THE
LOW POTASSIUM DIET
COOKBOOK

--------------------~----------------

85 Low Potassium & Healthy Homemade Recipes for People with High Potassium Levels in Blood (Hyperkalemia)

--------------------~----------------

ALSO INCLUDES: DETAILED NUTRITIONAL INFORMATION FOR EACH RECIPE

BY

MONIKA SHAH

COPYRIGHT © 2015

A Message for Readers!

Maintain Right Potassium Levels With Right Diet & Right Portions

This book has been specifically designed and written for people who have been diagnosed with high potassium levels in the blood (Hyperkalemia) or other similar medical conditions where they need to limit their intake of potassium.

Let's take a closer look on what this book has to offer:

- **The Low Potassium Diet Cookbook:** The cookbook has 85 Low potassium and healthy homemade recipes which are designed especially for people with high potassium levels in the blood or other similar medical conditions. The recipes in the book have been designed using very simple ingredients that people use in their kitchen every day or can find in the grocery stores very easily. These recipes are further categorized into **Main Dishes, Sides Dishes, Beverages and Desserts.**

- **Healthy & Delicious Recipes:** The whole purpose of these recipes is to make sure that the person with high potassium levels enjoys life without compromising the taste of the real food. Each recipe in this book has easy to find ingredients and steps with accurate serving sizes and detailed nutritional values. You will find recipes which can be eaten daily or on occasions without even compromising with health a bit.

- **Accurate Nutritional Information:** Each recipe comes with an accurate Nutritional Information Table to help people with high potassium levels know what nutrition they are getting and in what quantities. The nutritional table of each recipe provides "Amounts per serving" details for:

- *Calories*
- *Trans Fat*
- *Sodium*
- *Protein*
- *Cholesterol*
- *Potassium*
- *Total Fat*
- *Carbohydrates*
- *Phosphorus*
- *Saturated Fat*
- *Fiber*
- *Calcium*

CONTENTS

Copyright Notes & Disclaimer

This Page Has Been Left Blank Intentionally.

Chapter 1

Understanding Potassium (A Mineral & Electrolyte)

Potassium is a mineral that helps your nerves and muscles work the right way. It is also an electrolyte, a substance that is responsible for conducting electricity in the body. It is found in many foods that you eat and plays a crucial role in keeping your heartbeat regular and muscles working right. It also helps to control blood pressure.

It is the job of the kidneys to maintain a relative and constant balance of potassium in the body. The kidneys do this by excreting just enough amounts of potassium. In order to understand it better, let's assume if you eat a lot of potassium, the kidneys will start excreting more potassium to match its intake. On the other hand, if you eat a very less amount of potassium or there is not enough potassium in the body, the kidneys will excrete either very less or virtually no potassium to maintain the right balance of potassium in the body.

However, if your kidneys are not working the way they are supposed to, it is important that you limit or reduce the intake of foods that are known to increase the potassium level in your blood to an extreme dangerous level. When potassium level starts building in the blood, you may feel tingling, numbness and weakness. If the potassium in your body becomes too high, it may result in irregular heartbeats or even a heart attack.

Daily Recommended Intake of Potassium

In general, when you are healthy and your body organs, especially kidney are functioning the way they are supposed to, the recommended daily intake of potassium should be between 4500 – 5000 milligrams per day.

If you are suffering from Hyperkalemia or other similar medical conditions like Chronic Kidney Disease (CKD), kidneys are not able to remove enough potassium from the body and unable to maintain normal blood levels. In such case, you must limit the intake of potassium in your diet. In such condition, your daily potassium intake should not be more than 2000 to 3000 milligrams per day. It is better to limit it to between 2000 to 2500 milligrams per day.

Safe Levels of Potassium in Blood

The following table lists the various potassium levels in the body and their zones classifications.

Mmol/L	Zone
3.5-5.0	Safe
5.1-6.0	Caution
higher than 6.0	Danger

Chapter 2

How to Control & Lower High Potassium Levels

It is important to understand that most of the foods contain potassium, some in high amounts and some in less. It is you who need to decide on what to eat and how much. You can eat your favorite foods but must make sure that your daily recommended potassium levels are not exceeded. Eat the right and recommended portions and you will be absolutely fine.

If you have been diagnosed with high potassium levels in your blood and asked to limit its intake, then you must adhere to a low potassium diet, eat right and calculated portions as well as make sure that you follow the below listed tips to help reduce your potassium intake.

Tips to Reduce Potassium Intake

- Try to avoid salt and use the herbs and spices instead in the cooking and also at the dining table.
- Try not to use the substitutes of salt that are available in the market as they contain high amount of potassium and must be avoided.
- Some of the packaged foods like tomato products and canned soups contain potassium chloride that can be used in place of salt.

- You can eat a variety of foods but in moderation.
- It is advisable that you do not use or drink the juices from cooked meat and also the liquid from the canned vegetables and fruits.
- If you also have diabetes, you can choose to drink cranberry, grapes or apple juice when the blood sugar level in your body goes down.
- There is one important thing to remember that almost all foods have some amount of potassium. The size of the serving you eat is extremely important. For example, big amount or servings of a low potassium food can become a high-potassium food.
- It is also important that you leach the vegetables that are extremely high in potassium. Leaching is a process using which some amount of potassium can be pulled out of these high potassium vegetable.

Please refer to chapter 6 on "**Leaching Method to Reduce Potassium from Vegetables**".

Eat These Foods	Instead of These Foods
Cooked rice and wheat cereals	Bran cereals
White bread and pasta	Whole wheat bread and pasta
Rice milk (not enriched)	Cow's milk
White rice	Brown and wild rice

What to Look For On Food Labels

While buying food from supermarket or grocery stores, it is important to look at the nutritional values provided on the packaging. Please follow the guidelines provided below to measure the high and low potassium levels in the food.

- Foods that contain more than 15% of the DV (daily value) or 250 mg (milligrams) of potassium are considered as high in potassium.
- Foods that contain between 5 to 15% of the DV (daily value) or 121 to 250 mg (milligrams) of potassium are considered as medium in potassium.
- Foods that contain less than 5% of the DV (daily value) or less than 120 mg (milligrams) of potassium are considered as low in potassium.

This Page Has Been Left Blank Intentionally.

Chapter 3

Foods with High Potassium Levels

People who suffer from high potassium levels in their blood must know about the foods and food types that are high in potassium. It is important to know so that the consumption of such foods can either be avoided or reduced to accepted portions. Foods that contain more than 15% of the DV (daily value) or 250 mg (milligrams) of potassium are considered as high in potassium.

The following is the list of foods that are very high in potassium and must be avoided or limited.

Note: Though these foods are high in potassium but you can still enjoy some of these foods like chicken, red meat, milk, salmon etc. if you limit the intake to recommended potassium and one portion only. A list of foods that you should always avoid has been provided in Chapter 5.

Vegetables	Fruits
Acorn Squash	Apricot, raw
Artichoke	Apricot, dried
Bamboo Shoots	Avocado
Baked Beans	Banana
Butternut Squash	Cantaloupe
Refried Beans	Dates
Beets, fresh then boiled	Dried fruits
Black Beans	Figs, dried
Broccoli, cooked	Grapefruit Juice

Brussels Sprouts	Honeydew
Chinese Cabbage	Kiwi
Carrots, raw	Mango
Dried Beans and Peas	Nectarine
Greens, except Kale	Orange
Hubbard Squash	Orange Juice
Kohlrabi	Papaya
Lentils	Pomegranate
Legumes	Pomegranate Juice
White Mushrooms, cooked	Prunes
Okra	Prune Juice
Parsnips	Raisins
Potatoes, white and sweet	
Pumpkin	
Rutabagas	
Spinach, cooked	
Tomatoes	
Tomato products	
Vegetable Juices	

Other Foods

Bran/Bran products	Snuff/Chewing Tobacco
Chocolate	Cream
Granola	Red meats
Milk, all types	Chicken
Molasses	Salmon
Nuts and Seeds	Cod
Peanut Butter	Flounder
Salt Substitutes/Lite Salt	Sardines
Salt Free Broth	Scallops
Yogurt	

Chapter 4

Foods with Low Potassium Levels

Please remember that eating more than 1 portion can make a lower potassium food into a higher potassium food. Foods that contain less than 5% of the DV (daily value) or less than 120 mg (milligrams) of potassium are considered as low in potassium. Foods that contain between 5 to 15% of the DV (daily value) or 121 to 250 mg (milligrams) of potassium are considered as medium in potassium.

The following is the list of foods that are low in potassium and must be included in daily diet.

Vegetables	Fruits
Alfalfa sprouts	Apple
Asparagus	Apple Juice
Beans, green or wax	Applesauce
Cabbage, green and red Carrots, cooked	Apricots, canned in juice
Cauliflower	Blackberries
Celery	Blueberries
Corn, fresh	Cherries
Corn, frozen	Cranberries
Cucumber	Fruit Cocktail
Eggplant	Grapes
Kale	Grape Juice
Lettuce	Grapefruit
Mixed Vegetables	Mandarin Oranges

White Mushrooms, raw	Peaches, fresh
Onions	Peaches, canned
Parsley	Pears, fresh
Peas, green	Pears, canned
Peppers	Pineapple
Radish	Pineapple Juice
Rhubarb	Plums
Water Chestnuts, canned	Raspberries
Watercress	Strawberries
Yellow Squash	Tangerine
Zucchini Squash	Watermelon
Other Foods	
Rice	Eggs
Noodles	American cheese
Pasta	Cheddar cheese
Bread and bread products (Not Whole Grains)	Butter
Cake: angel, yellow	Cottage cheese
Coffee: limit to 8 ounces	Bagel
Pies without chocolate or high potassium fruit	Cider
Cookies without nuts or chocolate	Mayonnaise
Tea: limit to 16 ounces	Pickles
Vinegar	Honey

Chapter 5

Guidelines for Healthy Cooking

This chapter will help you with some of the standard yet important cooking guidelines that are extremely important not only for normal cooking but also for any health condition cooking too. These are basics of any kind of cooking but either people are not aware of these or do not care to follow them.

For any kind of health condition cooking, it is highly recommended that you read through each and every guideline carefully and apply them accordingly as and when required in your recipes and cooking.

How to Perfectly Measure and Weigh Ingredients

It is important for any kind of cooking that you measure your ingredients accurately. The measurement is even more important when you do cooking for certain health condition. This is required to maintain the right amount of nutrients and their nutritional values in the recipes.

The most important rules you must follow while using any cookbook are:

- Read every word of the recipe carefully.
- Make sure the measurements are accurate.

It is recommended that some sort of measuring tools are always kept in the kitchen so that they can be used as and when required. They can be of glass, plastic or even metal. Let's have a look below now what kind of measurement tools are best for measuring liquid and dry ingredients.

For liquid Ingredients

You can keep the liquid ingredients in the glass cups with pour spouts. While measuring liquid ingredients, you can simply place a cup on the flat surface and pour the liquid and read the desired mark at the eye level.

For dry ingredients

You can use individual cups in the sets of 1 cup, ½ cup, ⅓ cup and ¼ cup sizes. While measuring the dry ingredients, pile lightly into the measuring cup with spoon. Do not shake cup, level of with a straight edge.

Some Tips on measuring spoons:

- Measuring spoons are available in the sets of 1 tablespoon, 1 teaspoon, ½ teaspoon, ¼ teaspoon, and ⅛ teaspoon.
- Use for small amounts of dry foods or liquids.
- Dip spoon into dry ingredient, scoop, and then level of with a straight edge.
- Do not pour or level the ingredient over the bowl with the other ingredients.

Foods to Avoid & Their Healthy Substitutions

If you are just using this book as your guide for low potassium cooking then you may skip this chapter but if you take recipes from some other sources too, then you may need to know that there are certain foods that are not good for people with high potassium levels in blood.

The following is the list of foods that you should avoid eating or adding into your recipes with their healthy substitutes.

Food (Type)	Healthy Substitutes
Bouillon cubes	Homemade stock from cooked chicken or beef
Cakes mix	Homemade cakes
Garlic salt	Fresh or powdered garlic
Instant gravy/sauce mix	Thicken pan dripping with flour or corn starch
Instant rice and cereals	Long cooking rice and cereals (5 minutes or more)
Onion salt	Fresh or powdered onion
Salt	Spices and herbs
Self-rising cornmeal	Plain cornmeal plus baking powder
All-purpose flour (1 cup) plus baking	All-purpose flour (1 cup) plus baking powder (1 ½ tablespoon)
Worcestershire or soy sauce (1 teaspoon)	Liquid smoke (1 teaspoon)

Foods to Limit during High Potassium Levels

The following is the list of food that should be omitted from your recipes unless otherwise specified by your doctor or dietician/Nutritionist.

Apricots	Baking Soda
Bananas	Black-Eyed Peas
Bouillon Cubes	Cheese
Coconut	Cream Soups
Cream Style Corn	Dates
Dill Pickles	Instant Mixes
Instant Rice	Lima Beans
Mango	Melons
Monosodium Glutamate (MSG)	Nuts
Oranges	Orange Juice
Prunes	Raisins
Salt	Sweet Relish Pickles
Tomatoes	Tomato Juice
Tomato Sauce	Tomato Paste
Tomato Soup	Water Chestnuts

Note: The whole idea of a low potassium diet is to maintain the right potassium levels in the body by limiting its intake. You can do this by avoiding foods listed above and reducing the intake of some of the foods listed in chapter 3 to an acceptable level.

Alternate Healthy Seasonings & Usage Suggestions

Seasoning is an important part of cooking, especially salt but there are certain health conditions where salt adds to bad and poor health due to high sodium content levels. If you feel that the absence of salt decreases the flavor of food, try using herbs and spices to make up and bring that natural flavor of the food.

While using spices, use them in their dried form, either whole or ground whereas herbs can be in fresh or dried form. Spices and herbs are well known for enhancing the natural flavor of foods. In order to store them, spices and herbs should be stored in the cool and dry place in an airtight container. The airtight container will help retaining their freshness and flavors for a long time.

Let's have a look at the healthy seasoning alternates to salt and their appropriate uses below.

Herbs & Spices	Suggested Uses
ALLSPICE	Pot roast, fish, eggs, squash, fruit, relishes.
ANISE	Cookies, cakes, bread, candy, beverages, beef stew, stewed fruits, fish, shellfish.
BASIL	Noodles, rice, beef stew, pork, meat loaf, duck, fish, veal, salads, cooked vegetables, omelettes, dressings.
BAY LEAF	Soups, chowders, seafood, pot roast, stews.
BLACK PEPPER	Meats, poultry, fish, eggs, vegetables.

CARAWAY SEED	Green beans, beets, cabbage, carrots, cauliflower, zucchini, meat dishes/stews, marinades, cakes, cookies, rice, rye bread.
CARDAMON	Baked goods, grape jelly, puddings, squash, and fruit soups.
CELERY SEED	Salads, vegetables, stuffing's, breads, egg dishes, meat and fish dishes/stews, soups, marinades, dressings, dips.
CHILI POWDER	Barbecue sauces, dips, egg dishes, meat and chicken dishes, marinades.
CINNAMON	Baked goods, fruits, pork, ham, lamb, beef, chicken, hot beverages.
CLOVES	Fruits, baked goods, fish, meat sauces, pot roast, marinades, green beans, Harvard beets, carrots, stock, beverages.
CURRY POWDER	Meat, chicken, fish, eggs, dried beans, vegetables.
DILL SEED	Pickling, salads, soups, vegetables, fish, shellfish.
GARLIC	Soups, dips, sauces, salad dressings, dill pickles, meat, poultry, fish, stews, marinades, bread.
GINGER	Preserves, baked products, meat, poultry, fish, beverages, soups.
MACE	Baked goods, fruits, meat, fish, poultry, chowder, vegetables, and jellies.

MARJORAM	Meats, poultry, fish, game, sausages, stews, carrots, broccoli, pizza, spaghetti, eggplant, soup.
MINT	Punch, tea, desserts, sauce, jelly, fruit, edible garnish.
MUSTARD (DRY)	Egg and cheese dishes, salad dressings, meat, poultry, vegetables.
MUSTARD SEED	Coleslaw, boiled cabbage.
NUTMEG	Hot beverages, puddings, custards, baked goods, desserts, chicken, cream soups, seafood, eggs, vegetables.
ONION POWDER	Dips, soups, stews, all meats, fish, poultry, salads, vegetables, stuffing, egg dishes, breads, rice dishes.
OREGANO	Pasta dishes, pizza, barbecue sauce, vegetables, eggs, stuffing, pork, lamb, chicken, fish.
PAPRIKA	Meat, sausage, game, fish, poultry, egg dishes, vegetables, garnishing.
PARSLEY	Soups, meat sauces, stuffing, fish, meats, poultry, garnishing.
POPPY SEED	Pie crust, fruit compotes, fruit salad dressings, cookies, cakes, breads, garnishing.
POULTRY SEASONING	Stuffing, poultry, veal meat loaf, chicken soup.
RED PEPPER	Meats, soups, sauce, poultry, vegetables, spaghetti sauce,

	curried dishes, dips, tamale pie, barbecued beef and pork.
ROSEMARY	Lamb, poultry, veal, beef, pork, fish, soups, stews, marinades, stuffing, breads, dressings.
SAFFRON	Chicken, fish, seafood, soups, stews, rice.
SAGE	Stuffing, poultry, sauce, soups, fish, beef, pork, veal.
SESAME SEED	Edible garnish for salads, breads, meat dishes.
TARRAGON	Sauces, dressings, poultry, fish, egg dishes.
THYME	Meats, poultry, fish, stews, soups, vegetables.
TUMERIC	Curried meats, fish, poultry, egg dishes, colouring for cakes and rice dishes.
WHITE PEPPER	White sauces.

Chapter 6

Leaching Method to Reduce Potassium from Vegetables

Leaching is a process that helps in reducing potassium from high potassium vegetables to a great extent. Though, leaching does remove a great amount of potassium from vegetables but not in full. Keeping that in mind, it is still recommended that you limit the amount of leached high potassium vegetables in your diet.

The leaching process can be done for the following vegetables, especially root vegetables.

- Potatoes
- Sweet Potatoes
- Carrots
- Beets
- Winter Squash
- Rutabagas

In order to leach the above vegetables, please follow the below listed steps:

1. Start by peeling the vegetables. Once peeled, place them in cold water so that the vegetables won't become dark.
2. Next step is to slice the vegetables to 1/8th inches of thickness.
3. Now, for few seconds, rinse the vegetables in the warm water.

4. Now, soak the vegetables for about 2 hours in the warm water. For this process, you will have to use 10 times the amount of water of vegetables.
5. If you plan to soak the vegetables for a much longer duration than 2 hours, you must change the water every few hours.
6. Now, rinse the vegetables again under warm water.
7. While cooking, use 5 times the amount of water of vegetables to cook.

Chapter 7

Recipes: Main Dishes

A MESSAGE FOR READERS

This is important to understand that controlling your potassium intake is completely in your hands. In this chapter, you may see some recipes with more than 121-250 mg potassium per serving which is fine as you should only eat one portion of the recipe and a maximum of 2000 to 2500 milligrams of potassium per day. As long as your potassium intake is under the above mentioned limits, you will be fine.

Chicken Recipes

JALAPENO PEPPER CHICKEN

Yield: 8 servings

Serving size: 3-ounces

Ingredients

- 3 tablespoons vegetable oil
- 2-3 pounds chicken, cut up (skin and fat removed)
- 1 onion, sliced into rings
- 1 ½ cups homemade stock from cooked chicken
- ½ teaspoon ground nutmeg
- ¼ teaspoon black pepper
- 2 teaspoons fresh jalapeño peppers, finely chopped and seeded

Directions

- Start by heating the oil in a pan and brown the chicken pieces. Once the chicken pieces are brown, set them aside keeping warm.
- In the same pan, sauté the onion rings. Now, add the homemade stock from cooked chicken and bring to a boil. Keep stirring in between.
- Once the homemade stock from cooked chicken comes to a boil, add the chicken pieces, nutmeg and black pepper.
- Cover the pan the let the chicken simmer for 30 to 35 minutes or until the chicken is tender.
- Add jalapeño peppers to chicken and let it simmer for another minute or so. Serve hot.

Nutritional content per serving

Nutrition	Amount per serving
Calories	143
Trans Fat	0 grams
Sodium	45 milligrams
Protein	17 grams
Cholesterol	46 milligrams
Potassium	160 milligrams
Total Fat	7 grams
Carbohydrates	2 grams
Phosphorus	127 milligrams
Saturated Fat	1 gram
Fiber	0 grams
Calcium	12 milligrams

OVEN BROWN LEMON CHICKEN

Yield: 8 servings (or 8 pieces)

Serving size: 3 or 4-ounces

Ingredients

- 2 ½ pound fryer (cut as desired)
- 1 tablespoon lemon juice
- 1 cup all-purpose flour
- 1 teaspoon black pepper
- 1 cup corn flakes, crushed
- ¼ teaspoon poultry seasoning
- 4 tablespoons vegetable oil

Directions

- Start by preheating the oven to 400ºF.
- Next step is to wash, clean and pat dry the chicken pieces. Once the chicken pieces are dry, give them a bath of lemon juice.
- Take a small plastic bag and combine the flour, corn flakes, black pepper and poultry seasoning together. Shake the bag well to mix the ingredients.
- Take a deep baking pan (about 1 inch deep) and grease it with vegetable oil.
- Put the chicken in the plastic bag of ingredients and shake well. Put the large pieces first followed by small ones.
- Once the chicken pieces are well coated with the mixture, place them in the pan and brown in the oven for about 20 to 30 minutes on each side.

Nutritional content per serving

Nutrition	Amount per serving
Calories	280
Trans Fat	0 grams
Sodium	74 milligrams
Protein	15 grams
Cholesterol	52 milligrams
Potassium	150 milligrams
Total Fat	18 grams
Carbohydrates	15 grams
Phosphorus	120 milligrams
Saturated Fat	3 grams
Fiber	1 gram
Calcium	12 milligrams

OLD STYLE RICE AND CHICKEN

Yield: 6 servings

Serving size: ¾ cup

Ingredients

- 1 pound chicken parts
- 1 teaspoon black pepper
- 1 tablespoon poultry seasoning
- ½ cup chopped onion
- 1 teaspoon onion powder
- ½ teaspoon garlic powder
- 1 teaspoon crushed bay leaves (optional)
- 4 cups water
- 1 cup uncooked rice
- 1 tablespoon vegetable oil

Directions

- Take a Dutch oven covered with water and put the chicken pieces, spring onions, onion powder, black pepper, poultry seasoning and bay leaves.
- Cook the chicken until tender.
- Once the chicken is cooked, remove the chicken meat and skin from the bone. Keep the chicken meat but discard the skin. Also reserve 2 cups of chicken broth.
- Take a large pot and put rice, vegetable oil, chicken meat and 2 cups of chicken broth in it. Now, bring it to a boil over medium-high heat.

- Once it comes to a boil, reduce the heat to low and simmer for about 20 to 25 minutes.
- Serve hot.

Nutritional content per serving

Nutrition	Amount per serving
Calories	212
Trans Fat	0 grams
Sodium	76 milligrams
Protein	21 grams
Cholesterol	60 milligrams
Potassium	283 milligrams
Total Fat	8 grams
Carbohydrates	11 grams
Phosphorus	218 milligrams
Saturated Fat	2 grams
Fiber	1 gram
Calcium	25 milligrams

CHICKEN AND CELERY SALAD

Yield: 5 servings

Serving size: ¾ cup

Ingredients

- 2 cups chicken, diced
- 1/3 cup celery, chopped
- ¼ cup fresh onion, chopped
- ¼ cup fresh green pepper, chopped
- 1 teaspoon parsley, dried (optional)
- 1 tablespoon lemon juice
- ¼ teaspoon black pepper
- 1 teaspoon dry mustard
- ½ cup mayonnaise

Directions

- Take a bowl and combine chicken, parsley, celery, lemon juice and toss well.
- Take a small bowl and combine mustard, black pepper and mayonnaise together.
- Add the mustard mixture to chicken mixture and mix thoroughly

Nutritional content per serving

Nutrition	Amount per serving
Calories	181
Trans Fat	1 grams
Sodium	239 milligrams
Protein	18 grams
Cholesterol	47 milligrams
Potassium	205 milligrams
Total Fat	10 grams
Carbohydrates	3 grams
Phosphorus	149 milligrams
Saturated Fat	2 grams
Fiber	0 grams
Calcium	16 milligrams

SIMPLE VEGETABLES AND CHICKEN SALAD

Yield: 4 servings

Serving size: ½ cup

Ingredients

- 1 ½ cups cooked chicken, diced
- ½ cup green pepper, finely chopped
- ½ cup celery, finely diced
- ½ cup onions, finely chopped
- 3 tablespoons pimentos, diced
- ½ cup salad dressing or light mayonnaise
- 1 tablespoon lemon juice

Directions

- Take a bowl and combine chicken, spring onions, celery, and pimentos and toss well.
- Take a small bowl and combine lemon juice and mayonnaise.
- Add the mayonnaise mixture to chicken mixture and mix well.
- Cover and chill in the refrigerator before serving.

Nutritional content per serving

Nutrition	Amount per serving
Calories	221
Trans Fat	0 grams
Sodium	245 milligrams
Protein	18 grams
Cholesterol	47 milligrams
Potassium	230 milligrams
Total Fat	15 grams
Carbohydrates	15 grams
Phosphorus	143 milligrams
Saturated Fat	3 grams
Fiber	0 grams
Calcium	22 milligrams

SPRING ONIONS AND HERBS CHICKEN CURRY

Yield: 6 servings

Serving size: 3-ounces

Ingredients

- 1 whole chicken, skin removed, cut in small parts.
- ¼ cup lemon juice
- 2 teaspoons curry powder
- 1 medium onion, chopped
- 1 medium garlic glove, chopped (optional)
- ½ teaspoon black pepper
- ½ teaspoon dry thyme
- 2 tablespoon vegetable or olive oil
- 1 cup water

Directions

- Start by cleaning the whole chicken and cut into small pieces.
- Once you cut the chicken into small pieces, give the chicken pieces a bath of lemon juice.
- Next, take a medium sized bowl and combine spring onions, curry powder, black pepper, thyme together. Once combined, rub the mixture onto the chicken pieces.
- Next step is to let the chicken marinate in the refrigerator overnight or at least for 1 to 2 hours.

- Take a sauce pan and heat the vegetable oil. Sauté the marinated chicken until it turns brown.
- Once the chicken turns brown, pour one cup of water into the pan and let the chicken simmer until it gets tender.
- Once the chicken becomes tender, remove it from the heat and serve with hot rice.

Nutritional content per serving

Nutrition	Amount per serving
Calories	323
Trans Fat	0 grams
Sodium	93 milligrams
Protein	21 grams
Cholesterol	89 milligrams
Potassium	317 milligrams
Total Fat	24 grams
Carbohydrates	5 grams
Phosphorus	214 milligrams
Saturated Fat	6 grams
Fiber	0 grams
Calcium	25 milligrams

CHICKEN AND VEGETABLES STEW

Yield: 6 servings

Serving size: 1 cup

Ingredients

- 3 tablespoon vegetable oil
- 2 pounds chicken breast cut in bite size pieces
- 1 cup sliced onions
- ¾ cup green peppers
- 2 cloves garlic, minced
- 2 tablespoon all-purpose flour
- 2 10 ½-ounce cans low-sodium chicken broth
- 1 10-ounce bag frozen carrots
- ¼ teaspoon dried basil
- ¼ teaspoon black pepper
- 1 110-ounce bag frozen sliced okra

Directions

- Start by taking a Dutch oven and heating 2 tablespoons of oil in it.
- Now, add the chicken pieces and sauté the chicken over medium-high heat.
- Once the chicken is sautéed, remove it from the Dutch oven and set aside.
- Now, add 1 tablespoon of oil in the Dutch oven, add and sauté the onions, garlic and pepper.

- Now add the flour and cook it for about 2 to 3 minutes, stirring constantly.
- Now, add the chicken and broth and cook until it boils.
- Once the chicken broth comes to a boil, add the carrots, black pepper, and basil. Cover the Dutch oven and let it simmer for approximately 10 to 12 minutes. The gravy will become thick as it simmers.
- Now, add the okra and let it cook for another 5 to 10 minutes.
- Serve with hot white rice.

Nutritional content per serving

Nutrition	Amount per serving
Calories	142
Trans Fat	1 gram
Sodium	93 milligrams
Protein	10 grams
Cholesterol	15 milligrams
Potassium	453 milligrams
Total Fat	8 grams
Carbohydrates	13 grams
Phosphorus	129 milligrams
Saturated Fat	1 gram
Fiber	3 grams
Calcium	69 milligrams

Pork Recipes

SIMPLE 'N' BASIC PORK CHOPS

Yield: 4 chops

Serving size: 1 pork chop (3-ounces)

Ingredients

- 2 tablespoons vegetable oil
- ¼ cup all-purpose flour
- 1 teaspoon black pepper
- ½ teaspoon sage
- ½ teaspoon thyme
- 4 4-ounce lean pork chops (fat removed)

Directions

- Start by preheating the oven to 350ºF.
- Take a baking pan and grease it well with vegetable oil.
- Take a large bowl and combine the flour, thyme, sage and black pepper.
- Now dredge the pork chops in the flour mixture and arrange in the baking pan.
- Now place the baking pan into the oven and let the pork chops brown on both the sides. This process will take approximately 40-45 minutes.
- Once the pork chops are tender, remove them from the oven and serve hot.

Nutritional content per serving

Nutrition	Amount per serving
Calories	434
Trans Fat	0 grams
Sodium	60 milligrams
Protein	19 grams
Cholesterol	79 milligrams
Potassium	332 milligrams
Total Fat	34 grams
Carbohydrates	12 grams
Phosphorus	199 milligrams
Saturated Fat	10 grams
Fiber	0 grams
Calcium	35 milligrams

SIMPLE HOMEMADE PAN PORK SAUSAGE

Yield: 12 servings

Serving size: 1 patty

Ingredients

- 1 pound fresh lean ground pork, beef, chicken or turkey.
- 2 teaspoons ground sage
- 2 teaspoons granulated sugar
- 1 teaspoon ground black pepper
- ½ teaspoon ground red pepper
- 1 teaspoon basil (optional)
- Cooking spray

Directions

- Take a large bowl and mix all the ingredients well to make the sausage.
- Once the mixture is ready, make into patties by measuring 2 tablespoons of mixture for each patty.
- Once the patties are formed, either pan fry them or broil until they are thoroughly cooked.

Nutritional content per serving

Nutrition	Amount per serving
Calories	96
Trans Fat	0 grams
Sodium	22 milligrams
Protein	6 grams
Cholesterol	43 milligrams
Potassium	87 milligrams
Total Fat	7 grams
Carbohydrates	1 gram
Phosphorus	53 milligrams
Saturated Fat	2 grams
Fiber	0 grams
Calcium	72 milligrams

Lamb Recipes

GINGER & MUSTARD LAMB

Yield: 4 servings

Serving size: 3-ounces

Ingredients

- ¼ cup vegetable oil
- 1 ½ tablespoons garlic powder
- 3 teaspoons dry mustard
- 1 leg of lamb (trimmed for roasting)

Directions

- Start by taking a medium sized bowl and combining oil, mustard and ginger powder together well.
- Now, put and coat the lamb legs well with the mixture. Once the lamb legs are coated well with mixture, refrigerate the lamb legs for at least 6 to 8 hours or overnight.
- Remove the lamb from refrigerate and place on barbeque spit.
- Keep basting the meat continuously with the marinade and roast the lamb legs for around 30 minutes or until the meat thermometer reads the temperature of the lamb at 170 degrees F.

Nutritional content per serving

Nutrition	Amount per serving
Calories	289
Trans Fat	0 grams
Sodium	144 milligrams
Protein	24 grams
Cholesterol	73 milligrams
Potassium	423 milligrams
Total Fat	6 grams
Carbohydrates	3 grams
Phosphorus	237 milligrams
Saturated Fat	2 grams
Fiber	0 grams
Calcium	14 milligrams

Beef Recipes

BEEF 'N' RICE

Yield: 4 servings

Serving size: 1 cup

Ingredients

- 2 tablespoons vegetable oil
- 1 pound lean ground beef
- 1 cup onion, chopped
- 2 cups rice, cooked
- 1 ½ teaspoons chili con carne seasoning powder
- ⅛ teaspoon black pepper
- ½ teaspoon sage

Directions

- Start by heating the oil.
- Next step is to add the beef and onions. Cook the beef, stirring occasionally, until browns.
- Once the beef browns, add the rice, sage and chili con carne seasoning powder. Mix everything together well.
- Remove from the heat, cover and let stand for at least 10 to 15 minutes.

Nutritional content per serving

Nutrition	Amount per serving
Calories	360
Trans Fat	1 grams
Sodium	78 milligrams
Protein	23 grams
Cholesterol	65 milligrams
Potassium	27 milligrams
Total Fat	14 grams
Carbohydrates	26 grams
Phosphorus	233 milligrams
Saturated Fat	4 grams
Fiber	2 grams
Calcium	34 milligrams

PEPPERY BEEF STEAK

Yield: 4 servings

Serving size: 3-ounces

Ingredients

- 1 pound chopped steak or lean ground beef, chicken or turkey
- 1 small onion, chopped
- ½ cup green pepper, chopped
- 1 teaspoon black pepper
- 1 egg
- 1 tablespoon vegetable oil
- ½ cup water
- 1 tablespoon corn starch

Directions

- First step is to take a bowl and mix meat, green pepper, black pepper, onions and egg together well. Once mixed well, form the mixture into patties.
- Next step is to take a skillet and heat the oil. Once the oil is hot, place the patties in the skillet and cook on both the sides.
- Now, add half of half cup water and simmer for about 15 minutes. Remove the patties.
- Now, to the meat drippings, add the remaining water and corn starch. Let it simmer while constantly stirring to thicken the gravy.
- Final step is to pour the gravy over the steak and serve hot.

Nutritional content per serving

Nutrition	Amount per serving
Calories	249
Trans Fat	0 grams
Sodium	128 milligrams
Protein	22 grams
Cholesterol	149 milligrams
Potassium	366 milligrams
Total Fat	57 grams
Carbohydrates	7 grams
Phosphorus	218 milligrams
Saturated Fat	3 grams
Fiber	1 gram
Calcium	33 milligrams

HERBS BEEF BURGER

Yield: 4 servings

Serving size: 1 patty, 3-ounces

Ingredients

- 1 pound lean ground beef or ground turkey
- 1 tablespoon lemon juice
- 1 tablespoon parsley flakes
- ¼ teaspoon black pepper
- ¼ teaspoon ground thyme
- ¼ teaspoon oregano

Directions

- Start by mixing all the ingredients thoroughly in a medium or large bowl.
- Next step is to shape the mixture into patties. Please make the patties about ¾ inches thick.
- Now, take a skillet or broiler pan and grease it with a little oil.
- Final step is to broil the patties about 3 inches from the heat for about 10 to 15 minutes, turning once.

Nutritional content per serving

Nutrition	Amount per serving
Calories	171
Trans Fat	0 grams
Sodium	108 milligrams
Protein	20 grams
Cholesterol	90 milligrams
Potassium	289 milligrams
Total Fat	10 grams
Carbohydrates	0 grams
Phosphorus	180 milligrams
Saturated Fat	3 grams
Fiber	0 grams
Calcium	21 milligrams

HOMEMADE BEEF MEATBALLS

Yield: 35 meatballs

Serving size: 2 meatballs

Ingredients for meatballs

- 1 pound lean ground beef or turkey
- ¼ cup onions, finely chopped
- 1 tablespoon lemon juice
- 1 teaspoon poultry seasoning (without salt)
- 1 teaspoon black pepper
- ¼ teaspoon dry mustard
- ¾ teaspoon onion powder
- 1 teaspoon Italian seasoning
- 1 teaspoon granulated sugar
- 1 teaspoon Tabasco® sauce

Directions for meatballs

- Start by preheating the oven to 425ºF.
- Next step is to take a bowl and mix all the ingredients together well.
- Once the mixture is ready, shape the meatballs. Each meatball should have one tablespoon of meat mixture.
- Now, place the meatballs in a baking dish and bake them for about 20 minutes or until well done.
- Final step is to remove the meatballs from the oven and combine them with the sauce. Keep the meatballs warm until you are ready to serve.

Ingredients for sauce

- ¼ cup vegetable oil
- 2 tablespoons all-purpose flour
- 1 teaspoon onion powder
- 2 teaspoons vinegar
- 2 teaspoons sugar
- 1 teaspoon Tabasco® sauce
- 2-3 cups water

Directions for sauce

- Start by taking a sauce pan, placing on heat and combining oil and flour in it. Keep stirring.
- Now, add vinegar, sugar, onion powder, mild sauce and water
- Once you add all the ingredients, return the pan to heat and continue stirring until the sauce thickens.

Nutritional content per serving

Nutrition	Amount per serving
Calories	76
Trans Fat	0 grams
Sodium	31 milligrams
Protein	5 grams
Cholesterol	21 milligrams
Potassium	70 milligram
Total Fat	6 grams
Carbohydrates	2 grams
Phosphorus	44 milligrams
Saturated Fat	1 grams
Fiber	0 grams
Calcium	7 milligrams

BEEF STEAK SANDWICH

Yield: 4 servings

Serving size: 3-ounces

Ingredients

- 4 chopped steaks (4-ounces each)
- 1 tablespoon lemon juice
- 1 tablespoon Italian seasoning
- 1 tablespoon black pepper
- 1 tablespoon vegetable oil
- 1 medium onion, sliced into rings
- 4 hoagie rolls, sliced

Directions

- Start by taking a bowl and combining the meat, Italian seasoning, black pepper and lemon juice in it.
- Next step is to take a frying pan and heat the oil over medium heat.
- Next step is to brown the beef steaks on both the sides until they are tender. Once done, remove from the pan and drain on the paper towels.
- Now, reduce the heat and in the same pan, add onions and sauté them until they are tender.
- In order to serve, serve open faced on roasted or grilled bread slices.

Nutritional content per serving

Nutrition	Amount per serving
Calories	345
Trans Fat	0 grams
Sodium	247 milligrams
Protein	14 grams
Cholesterol	40 milligrams
Potassium	200 milligrams
Total Fat	21 grams
Carbohydrates	26 grams
Phosphorus	115 milligrams
Saturated Fat	7 grams
Fiber	2 grams
Calcium	98 milligrams

BEEF TACOS

Yield: 8 servings

Serving size: 2-ounces stuffing in each shell

Ingredients

- 2 tablespoon vegetable oil
- 1 ¼ pounds lean ground beef or turkey
- ½ teaspoon ground red pepper
- ½ teaspoon black pepper
- 1 teaspoon Italian seasoning
- 1 teaspoon garlic powder
- 1 teaspoons onion powder
- ½ teaspoon Tabasco® sauce
- ½ teaspoon nutmeg
- 1 medium taco shells
- ½ head shredded lettuce

Directions

- Start by taking a skillet and heating oil.
- Next step is to place the meat and all other ingredients except the tack shells and lettuce in the skillet.
- Next, cook the beef until done and all ingredients are well blended.
- Final step is to stuff the taco shells with 2 ounces of meat and top it with the shredded lettuce.

Nutritional content per serving

(Inclusive of taco shells and shredded lettuce)

Nutrition	Amount per serving
Calories	176 calories
Trans Fat	0 grams
Sodium	124 milligrams
Protein	14 grams
Cholesterol	56 milligrams
Potassium	258 milligrams
Total Fat	9 grams
Carbohydrates	9 grams
Phosphorus	150 milligrams
Saturated Fat	2 grams
Fiber	0 grams
Calcium	33 milligrams

Turkey Recipes

SIMPLE 'N' BASIC TURKEY MEAT LOAF

Yield: 8 servings

Serving size: 2-ounces

Ingredients

- 1 pound lean ground turkey
- 1 egg white
- 1 tablespoon lemon juice
- ½ cup plain bread crumbs
- ½ teaspoon onion powder
- ½ teaspoon Italian seasoning
- ¼ teaspoon black pepper
- ½ cup chopped onions
- ½ cup diced green bell pepper
- ¼ cup water

Directions

- Start by preheating the oven to 400ºF.
- Place the meat in a bowl and pour lemon juice on it.
- Add all other remaining ingredients to meat and mix well.
- Finally, place the loaf in a pan and bake for about 45 minutes.

Nutritional content per serving

Nutrition	Amount per serving
Calories	110
Trans Fat	0 grams
Sodium	71 milligrams
Protein	12 grams
Cholesterol	42 milligrams
Potassium	138 milligrams
Total Fat	5 grams
Carbohydrates	2 grams
Phosphorus	87 milligrams
Saturated Fat	1 grams
Fiber	0 grams
Calcium	20 milligram

Seafood Recipes

FISH CROQUETTES

Yield: 8 patties

Serving size: 1 patty

Ingredients

- 1 can water packed salmon or tuna (14.75-ounce), or 1 pound frozen or fresh crab meat.
- 2 egg whites
- ¼ cup chopped onion
- ½ teaspoon black pepper
- ½ cup plain bread crumb or unsalted cracker crumbs
- 1 tablespoon vegetable oil or cooking spray
- 2 tablespoons lemon juice (optional)
- ½ teaspoon ground mustard (crab only)
- ¼ cup regular mayonnaise (tuna and crab only)

Directions

- Start by draining the water from the canned meat.
- Next step is to take a medium bowl and combine all the ingredients except oil and mix well.
- Once the mixture is mixed well, form the mixture into 8 separate balls, and then flatten them to form patties.
- Next step is to take a skillet and heat vegetable oil in it.
- Once the oil is hot, place the patties in it.
- Brown the patties on each side. Once the patties are cooked, drain them on paper towels.

Nutritional content per serving

Nutrition	Amount per serving
Calories	189
Trans Fat	0 grams
Sodium	337 milligrams
Protein	14 grams
Cholesterol	81 milligrams
Potassium	184 milligrams
Total Fat	8 grams
Carbohydrates	11 grams
Phosphorus	191 milligrams
Saturated Fat	2 grams
Fiber	1 gram
Calcium	124 milligrams

BAKED TROUT FILLETS

Yield: 4 servings

Serving size: 3-ounces

Ingredients

- 4 3-ounce trout filets or any other baking fish
- 1 ½ teaspoon black pepper
- 1 tablespoon garlic powder
- 1 ½ teaspoon paprika
- ¼ medium green pepper
- 1 small onion
- 1 small lemon

Directions

- Start by preheating the oven to 375ºF.
- Next step is to place the fish in a greased baking pan or on aluminum foil.
- Now sprinkle the garlic powder, black pepper, and paprika on both sides of the fish.
- Also place the chopped spring onions on fish.
- Now, squeeze the juice of one lemon onto fish.
- It's now time to bake the fish for 30 minutes.
- After the fish has cooked, sprinkle with parmesan cheese.
- Serve hot.

Nutritional content per serving

Nutrition	Amount per serving
Calories	164
Trans Fat	0 grams
Sodium	86 milligrams
Protein	20 grams
Cholesterol	62 milligrams
Potassium	452 milligrams
Total Fat	6 grams
Carbohydrates	8 grams
Phosphorus	252 milligrams
Saturated Fat	1 grams
Fiber	3 grams
Calcium	80 milligrams

SHRIMPS & EGGS SALAD

Yield: 4 servings

Serving size: ½ cup

Ingredients

- 1 pound shrimp, boiled, chopped and deveined
- 1 hard-boiled egg, chopped
- 1 tablespoon celery, chopped
- 1 tablespoon green pepper, chopped
- 1 tablespoon onion, chopped
- 2 tablespoons mayonnaise
- 1 teaspoon lemon juice
- ½ teaspoon chili powder
- ⅛ teaspoon Tabasco® or hot sauce
- ½ teaspoon dry mustard
- Lettuce, chopped or shredded (optional)

Directions

- Start by combining all the ingredients except lettuce, in a mixing bowl. Mix well.
- Chill the mixture in the refrigerator for about 30 minutes.
- To serve: serve as a salad over a bed of lettuce, if desired, or serve on a sandwich.

Nutritional content per serving

Nutrition	Amount per serving
Calories	157
Trans Fat	0 grams
Sodium	232 milligrams
Protein	26 grams
Cholesterol	234 milligrams
Potassium	233 milligrams
Total Fat	5 grams
Carbohydrates	1 gram
Phosphorus	263 milligrams
Saturated Fat	1 grams
Fiber	0 grams
Calcium	67 milligrams

SUPREME OF SHRIMPS & CRABS

Yield: 6 servings

Serving size: ½ cup

Ingredients

- 1 cup crabmeat, cooked (boiled)
- 1 cup shrimp, cooked (boiled)
- 4 tablespoons green pepper, chopped
- 2 tablespoons green onions, chopped
- 1 cup celery, chopped
- ½ cup frozen green peas
- ½ teaspoon black pepper
- ½ cup mayonnaise
- 1 cup bread crumbs

Directions

- Start by preheating the oven to 375ºF.
- Combine all the ingredients except the bread crumbs in a bowl.
- Now, place the mix in a greased casserole dish and top with bread crumbs.
- Finally, bake it for about 30 minutes.

Nutritional content per serving

Nutrition	Amount per serving
Calories	220
Trans Fat	0 grams
Sodium	445 milligrams
Protein	16 grams
Cholesterol	28 milligrams
Potassium	255 milligrams
Total Fat	8 grams
Carbohydrates	20 grams
Phosphorus	148 milligrams
Saturated Fat	1 gram
Fiber	2 grams
Calcium	85 milligrams

BAKED LEMON CRAB CAKES

Yield: 6 servings

Serving size: 1 patty

Ingredients

- 1 egg (egg substitute or egg white optional)
- 1/3 cup green or red pepper, finely chopped
- 1/3 cup low sodium crackers
- ¼ cup reduced fat mayonnaise
- 1 tablespoon dry mustard
- 1 teaspoon crushed red pepper or black pepper
- 2 tablespoons lemon juice
- 1 teaspoon garlic powder
- 2 tablespoon vegetable oil

Directions

- Start by combining all ingredients.
- Now, divide the mixture into 6 balls and form patties.
- Take a pan and heat vegetable oil at medium heat or oven at 350ºF.
- Fry the patties for about 4-5 minutes or bake in the oven for 15 minutes.
- Serve warm.

Nutritional content per serving

Nutrition	Amount per serving
Calories	101
Trans Fat	0 grams
Sodium	67 milligrams
Protein	2 grams
Cholesterol	41 milligrams
Potassium	72 milligrams
Total Fat	9 grams
Carbohydrates	5 grams
Phosphorus	43 milligrams
Saturated Fat	1 gram
Fiber	0 grams
Calcium	16 milligrams

BAKED FLAKY FISH FILLETS

Yield: 4 servings

Serving size: 3 ½-ounces

Ingredients

- 12-16 fish filets (1 pound), tilapia or as desired
- 20 saltine crackers, unsalted tops, crushed finely
- ¼ cup unsalted butter or margarine
- 2 teaspoon dill weed
- 1 teaspoon garlic powder
- ¼ cup lemon juice

Directions

- Start by preheating the oven to 400ºF.
- Now, combine the dill, crackers and garlic powder.
- Next, melt the butter or margarine.
- Now, roll the fish in the melted butter, then in crumbs and again in the butter mix.
- Finally, place in the baking pan and bake for about 8 to 10 minutes until the fish is flaky.

Nutritional content per serving

Nutrition	Amount per serving
Calories	164
Trans Fat	0 grams
Sodium	138 milligrams
Protein	21 grams
Cholesterol	57 milligrams
Potassium	335 milligrams
Total Fat	6 grams
Carbohydrates	7 grams
Phosphorus	181 milligrams
Saturated Fat	4 grams
Fiber	0 grams
Calcium	23 milligrams

ROTINI 'N' TUNA

Yield: 4 servings

Serving size: 1 cup

Ingredients

- Vegetable cooking spray
- 2 tablespoons minced fresh onion
- 2/3 cup water
- ¼ teaspoon curry powder
- ¼ teaspoon black pepper
- 1 10 ¾-ounce can low sodium cream of mushroom soup, undiluted
- 2 cups hot cooked rotini (corkscrew pasta, cooked without salt or fat)
- ½ cup frozen green peas, thawed
- 1 9 ¼-ounce low sodium albacore tuna, with water, drained
- Chopped fresh parsley (optional)

Directions

- Take a large non-stick skillet and coat it with cooking spray. Place the skillet over medium heat.
- Now, add onions and sauté them until they are tender.
- Now, take a bowl and combine water, pepper, curry powder and soup. Stir well and then add to skillet.
- Now, add cooked tuna, rotini and peas. Stir well.
- Let it cook uncovered over low heat for about 10 minutes, stirring occasionally.

- Sprinkle with parsley, if desired.

Nutritional contents per serving

Nutrition	Amount per serving
Calories	269
Trans Fat	0 gram
Sodium	407 milligrams
Protein	18 grams
Cholesterol	58 milligrams
Potassium	515 milligrams
Total Fat	4 grams
Carbohydrates	38 grams
Phosphorus	228 milligrams
Saturated Fat	0 gram
Fiber	1 gram
Calcium	30 milligrams

Soup Recipes

BEEF & VEGETABLES SOUP

Yield: 8 servings

Serving size: ¾ cup

Ingredients

- 1 pound beef stew
- 3 ½ cups water
- 1 cup raw sliced onions
- ½ cup frozen green peas
- 1 teaspoon black pepper
- ½ cup frozen okra
- ½ teaspoon basil
- ½ cup frozen carrots, diced
- ½ teaspoon thyme
- ½ cup frozen corn

Directions

- Take a large pot and place beef stew, black pepper, onions, basil, thyme and water. Let cook for about 45 minutes.
- Now, add all frozen vegetables. Simmer it on low heat until the meat is tender. If additional water is needed in the soup, you may add ½ cup at a time.
- Serve hot.

Nutritional content per serving

Nutrition	Amount per serving
Calories	190
Trans Fat	0 grams
Sodium	56 milligrams
Protein	11 grams
Cholesterol	42 milligrams
Potassium	291 milligrams
Total Fat	13 grams
Carbohydrates	7 grams
Phosphorus	121 milligrams
Saturated Fat	5 grams
Fiber	2 grams
Calcium	31 milligrams

EGG NOODLES & CHICKEN SOUP

Yield: 8 servings

Serving size: ¾ cup

Ingredients

- 1 pound chicken parts
- 1 teaspoon red pepper
- ¼ cup lemon juice
- 1 teaspoon caraway seed
- 3 ½ cups water
- 1 teaspoon oregano
- 1 tablespoon poultry seasoning
- 1 teaspoon sugar
- 1 teaspoon garlic powder
- ½ cup celery
- 1 teaspoon onion powder
- ½ cup green pepper
- 2 tablespoons vegetable oil
- 1 cup egg noodles
- 1 teaspoon black pepper

Directions

- Start by rubbing the chicken parts with lemon juice.
- Take a large pot and combine the chicken, water, garlic powder, poultry seasoning, black pepper, onion powder, vegetable oil, caraway seed, oregano, red pepper and sugar together.

- Let cook for about 30 minutes or until the chicken is tender.
- Add the remaining ingredients and cook for additional 15 minutes. If additional water is needed in the soup, you may add ½ cup at a time.
- Serve hot.

Nutritional content per serving

Nutrition	Amount per serving
Calories	110
Trans Fat	0 grams
Sodium	17 milligrams
Protein	3 grams
Cholesterol	12 milligrams
Potassium	101 milligrams
Total Fat	8 grams
Carbohydrates	7 grams
Phosphorus	39 milligrams
Saturated Fat	2 grams
Fiber	0 grams
Calcium	21 milligrams

Egg Recipes

HERBACEOUS OMELETTE

Yield: 2 servings

Serving size: ½ omelet

Ingredients

- 1 ½ teaspoons vegetable oil
- 1 tablespoon chopped onion
- 4 eggs
- 2 tablespoons water
- ¼ teaspoon basil
- ⅛ teaspoon tarragon
- ¼ teaspoon parsley (optional)

Directions

- Take a bowl and beat the eggs. Now, add water and spices.
- Now, heat the oil in an 8" frying pan over medium heat. Once the oil is hot, add and sauté the spring onions. Remove from the pan.
- Now, pour the mixture into heated frying pan over medium heat.
- As the omelette sets, lift with the help of a spatula to let the uncooked portion of the omelette flow to the bottom.
- When the omelette is completely set, add the sautéed spring onions to the top of the omelette and remove from pan to a serving dish.

Nutritional content per serving

Nutrition	Amount per serving
Calories	195
Trans Fat	0 grams
Sodium	157 milligrams
Protein	14 grams
Cholesterol	474 milligrams
Potassium	157 milligrams
Total Fat	15 gram
Carbohydrates	0 grams
Phosphorus	214 milligrams
Saturated Fat	4 grams
Fiber	0 grams
Calcium	60 milligrams

FRUITY OMELETTE

Yield: 4 servings

Serving size: ¼ omelet

Ingredients

- 2 cups frozen unsweetened strawberries, thawed
- 1 tablespoon sugar (optional)
- 4 eggs, separated
- 1 tablespoon lemon juice
- 1 tablespoon unsalted butter or margarine

Directions

- Start by preheating the oven to 375ºF.
- Now, sprinkle thawed strawberries with sugar, keep aside and let stand.
- Take a medium bowl and beat the egg whites until stiff
- Take a separate bowl and beat the egg yolks and lemon juice. Now, fold the stiff beaten egg whites into the beaten yolks until no yellow streaks remain.
- Take a 10" skillet that is oven-safe and melt butter in it. Pour the egg mixture into the skillet, tilting pan to coat sides. Let cook over low heat for about 5 minutes.
- When the mixture is set on the bottom, cook in the oven for additional 5 minutes.
- Now, lift the omelette onto heated plate. Spoon on strawberries and cut into pie wedges.
- Serve hot.

Nutritional content per serving

Nutrition	Amount per serving
Calories	198
Trans Fat	0 grams
Sodium	125 milligrams
Protein	8 grams
Cholesterol	240 milligrams
Potassium	430 milligrams
Total Fat	9 grams
Carbohydrates	24 grams
Phosphorus	141 milligrams
Saturated Fat	4 grams
Fiber	7 grams
Calcium	56 milligrams

Miscellaneous Recipes

MEAT STUFFED GREEN PEPPERS

Yield: 6 servings

Serving size: 1 stuffed pepper

Ingredients

- 2 tablespoon vegetable oil
- ½ pound ground lean beef, turkey or chicken
- ¼ cup onions, chopped
- ¼ cup celery, chopped
- 2 tablespoons lemon juice
- 1 tablespoon celery seed
- 2 tablespoons Italian seasoning
- 1 teaspoon black pepper
- ½ teaspoon sugar
- 1 ½ cup of cooked rice
- 6 small green peppers, seeded with tops removed
- Paprika

Directions

- Start by preheating the oven to 325ºF.
- Take a saucepan and heat oil in it.
- Now, add the ground meat, celery and onions to pan, cook together until the meat is browned.
- Now, add all the ingredients except the paprika and green peppers to the sauce pan. Stir together and remove from the heat.
- Stuff the peppers with mixture.

- Finally, wrap with the foil or place the peppers in a dish and cover. Bake the peppers for about 30 minutes. Once done, remove from the oven and sprinkle with paprika.

Nutritional content per serving

Nutrition	Amount per serving
Calories	131
Trans Fat	0 grams
Sodium	36 milligrams
Protein	9 grams
Cholesterol	28 milligrams
Potassium	160 milligrams
Total Fat	4 grams
Carbohydrates	15 grams
Phosphorus	83 milligrams
Saturated Fat	1 gram
Fiber	1 gram
Calcium	38 milligrams

MEAT EGGPLANT CASSEROLE

Yield: 8 servings

Serving size: ½ cup

Ingredients

- 1 large eggplant
- 2 tablespoon vegetable oil
- ½ cup green pepper, chopped
- ½ cup onion, finely chopped
- 1 pound lean ground beef or turkey
- 2 cups plain bread crumbs
- 1 large egg, slightly beaten
- ½ teaspoon red pepper, optional

Directions

- Start by preheating the oven to 350ºF.
- Next step is to boil the eggplant until its tender. Once done, drain and mash the eggplant.
- Next step is to heat the oil in a pan. Once the oil is hot add onion, green pepper and ground meat. Sauté everything together until cooked.
- Now, add the eggplant, egg and bread crumbs. Mix well.
- Now, add the red pepper as per taste, if desired.
- Finally, bake in a casserole dish for about 30 to 45 minutes.
- Serve warm.

Nutritional content per serving

Nutrition	Amount per serving
Calories	240
Trans Fat	0 grams
Sodium	263 milligrams
Protein	15 grams
Cholesterol	74 milligrams
Potassium	380 milligrams
Total Fat	9 grams
Carbohydrates	5 grams
Phosphorus	169 milligrams
Saturated Fat	2 grams
Fiber	4 grams
Calcium	71 milligrams

STIR FRY VEGETABLES & CHICKEN

Yield: 3 servings

Serving size: ½ cup chicken and vegetables with 2/3 cup rice

Ingredients

- 2 tablespoon cooking oil
- 2 medium chicken breasts cut into bite size pieces
- 1 10-ounce package frozen stir fry vegetables
- ½ tablespoon liquid smoke
- 2 cups cooked rice

Directions

- Take 9 to 10 inches and heat the oil on high heat.
- Add the chicken, and sauté.
- Stir in the vegetables.
- Add the liquid smoke and stir everything well.
- Reduce the heat to medium high and let it cook uncovered for about 3 to 5 minutes, or until done, stirring frequently.
- Serve over 2/3 cup of cooked rice.

Nutritional content per serving

Nutrition	Amount per serving
Calories	315
Trans Fat	0 grams
Sodium	37 milligrams

Protein	29 grams
Cholesterol	76 milligrams
Potassium	618 milligrams
Total Fat	7 grams
Carbohydrates	32 grams
Phosphorus	26 milligrams
Saturated Fat	2 grams
Fiber	3 grams
Calcium	32 milligrams

CHICKEN 'N' RICE DRESSING

Yield: 4 servings

Serving size: 1 cup

Ingredients

- 2 tablespoons vegetable oil
- ¼ cup green peppers, chopped
- 1 pound lean ground turkey
- ½ teaspoon cayenne pepper
- 2 tablespoons all-purpose flour
- 1 clove garlic, chopped
- ¼ cup onion, chopped
- 2 cups hot cooked rice
- ¼ cup green onions, chopped
- 1 cup low sodium chicken broth (Try to use homemade)
- ¼ cup celery, chopped

Directions

- Start by preheating the oven to 350ºF.
- Take a skillet and heat the oil. Once the oil is hot, add the meat and let cook on medium heat until the meat is browned.
- Remove the meat from heat and drain on paper towels.
- Take another skillet and add flour. Brown the flour to make a dark roux.
- Now, add celery, onions, garlic and peppers to the roux and cook until the vegetables are tender.
- Now, add the cooked rice and the meat.

- Next step is to add the low sodium chicken broth a little at a time until mixture becomes moist. If the mixture is too dry, you may add some more water.
- Next, pour the mixture into a 1 ½ quart baking dish.
- Finally, bake it for about 20 minutes.

Nutritional content per serving

Nutrition	Amount per serving
Calories	393
Trans Fat	0 grams
Sodium	113 milligrams
Protein	27 grams
Cholesterol	84 milligrams
Potassium	377 milligrams
Total Fat	19 grams
Carbohydrates	28 grams
Phosphorus	228 milligrams
Saturated Fat	4 grams
Fiber	1 grams
Calcium	43 milligrams

CHICKEN FAJITAS

Yield: 4 servings

Serving size: 4 medium strips

Ingredients

- 2 tablespoon vegetable oil
- 1 ½ pounds raw chicken strips or beef strips or shrimp (peeled and deveined)
- 2 teaspoon chili powder
- ½ teaspoon cumin
- 2 tablespoon lemon or lime juice
- ¼ green and/or red pepper, sliced lengthwise
- ½ onion white, sliced lengthwise
- ½ teaspoon dry cilantro
- 4 flour tortillas
- Vegetable spray

Directions

- Start by preheating the oven to 300ºF.
- Take a non-stick frying pan and heat the vegetable oil over medium heat.
- Now, add the meat, lemon/lime juice, and seasonings. Cook for about 5 to 10 minutes or until the meat is tender.
- Now, add onion and pepper to the pan and cook for about 1 to 2 minutes.
- Remove the pan from heat and sprinkle cilantro.

- Take a foil and place tortillas on it and move to the oven. Just heat them for about 10 minutes
- Finally, divide the mixture between tortillas, wrap and serve.

Nutritional content per serving

Nutrition	Amount per serving
Calories	184
Trans Fat	0 grams
Sodium	121 milligrams
Protein	19 grams
Cholesterol	57 milligrams
Potassium	494 milligrams
Total Fat	10 grams
Carbohydrates	5 grams
Phosphorus	207 milligrams
Saturated Fat	1 gram
Fiber	1 gram
Calcium	38 milligrams

Chapter 8

Recipes: Sides Dishes

A MESSAGE FOR READERS

This is important to understand that controlling your potassium intake is completely in your hands. In this chapter, you may see some recipes with more than 121-250 mg potassium per serving which is fine as you should only eat one portion of the recipe and a maximum of 2000 to 2500 milligrams of potassium per day. As long as your potassium intake is under the above mentioned limits, you will be fine.

Breads & Starches Recipes

WHITE RICE O'BRIEN

Yield: 4 servings

Serving size: ½ cup

Ingredients

- 1½ cup water
- 1 cup rice, uncooked
- ½ cup onion, thinly sliced or chopped
- ¼ cup green pepper, chopped
- ¼ cup carrots, shredded
- ¼ teaspoon red pepper
- ½ teaspoon black pepper
- ½ teaspoon thyme or rosemary
- 1 tablespoon lemon juice
- 1 tablespoon margarine

Directions

- Take a large saucepan and boil water in it. In the boiling water, combine all ingredients.
- Cover the pan and let it simmer for about 15 minutes without stirring.
- Now, remove from the pan and fluff the rice lightly with the help of a fork.

Nutritional content per serving

Nutrition	Amount per serving
Calories	207
Trans Fat	1 gram
Sodium	32 milligrams
Protein	4 grams
Cholesterol	0 milligrams
Potassium	125 milligrams
Total Fat	3 grams
Carbohydrates	40 grams
Phosphorus	64 milligrams
Saturated Fat	1 grams
Fiber	1 grams
Calcium	21 milligrams

HERBACEOUS BREAD

Yield: 1 loaf — about 15 slices

Serving size: 1 slice

Ingredients

- 1 loaf French bread
- ¼ cup margarine (unsalted)
- 2 tablespoons chopped green onions
- 1 teaspoon thyme
- ¼ teaspoon tarragon
- 1 teaspoon basil flakes (optional)
- ½ teaspoon crushed marjoram (optional)

Directions

- Start by preheating the oven to 350ºF.
- Next, slice the French bread almost to the bottom crust.
- Take a bowl and combine margarine with the remaining ingredients.
- Now, spread the butter mixture onto the cut slices. You may use a brush for this purpose, if needed.
- Place the slices on a baking sheet and bake for about 15 to 20 minutes.

Nutritional content per serving

Nutrition	Amount per serving
Calories	120
Trans Fat	0 grams
Sodium	208 milligrams
Protein	4 grams
Cholesterol	0 milligrams
Potassium	44 milligrams
Total Fat	4 grams
Carbohydrates	18 grams
Phosphorus	37 milligrams
Saturated Fat	1 gram
Fiber	1 gram
Calcium	15 milligrams

FRESH BLUEBERRY BREAD

Yield: 6 servings

Serving size: ½ cup

Ingredients

- 1 quart blueberries, fresh or frozen
- ¼ cup water (omit if berries are frozen)
- 1 teaspoon lemon juice
- ½ cup sugar
- 1 pinch nutmeg
- 1 pinch cinnamon
- 1 tablespoon margarine
- 3 slices bread, buttered and sprinkled with cinnamon and sugar on both sides

Directions

- Start by preheating the oven to 425ºF.
- Next step is to wash the blueberries thoroughly under cool running water.
- Take a sauce pan and combine all the ingredients except the bread. Bring it to a boil.
- Now, pour the blueberry mixture into a shallow baking pan. Top the mixture with bread cut in halves.
- Finally, bake until it turns brown. This will take about 10 minutes.

Nutritional content per serving

Nutrition	Amount per serving
Calories	176
Trans Fat	0 grams
Sodium	92 milligrams
Protein	2 grams
Cholesterol	0 milligrams
Potassium	83 milligrams
Total Fat	3 grams
Carbohydrates	39 grams
Phosphorus	20 milligrams
Saturated Fat	0 grams
Fiber	3 grams
Calcium	56 milligrams

BLUEBERRY MUFFINS

Yield: 12 muffins

Serving size: 1 muffin

Ingredients

- 1 egg white
- ¼ cup margarine
- ½ cup sugar
- 7 tablespoons water
- ½ teaspoon vanilla extract
- 1 teaspoon baking powder
- 1 cup all-purpose flour
- 1 cup blueberries, canned and drained or fresh

Directions

- Start by preheating the oven to 375ºF.
- Take a small bowl and beat egg white until its stiff. Once done, keep it aside.
- Take another bowl and cream the margarine and sugar together until smooth.
- Now, add vanilla and water. Mix thoroughly.
- Now, add the flour and baking powder.
- Fold in the blueberries and beaten egg white.
- Finally, bake it in a greased muffin pan for about 30 minutes.

Nutritional content per serving

Nutrition	Amount per serving
Calories	123
Trans Fat	0 grams
Sodium	139 milligrams
Protein	1. 5 grams
Cholesterol	0 milligrams
Potassium	71 milligrams
Total Fat	4 grams
Carbohydrates	21 grams
Phosphorus	94 milligrams
Saturated Fat	0 gram
Fiber	1 gram
Calcium	29 milligrams

SIMPLY BISCUITS

Yield: 10 biscuits

Serving size: 1 biscuit

Ingredients

- 2 cups all-purpose flour, sifted
- 3 teaspoons double acting baking powder
- 2 teaspoons sugar
- ⅓ cup vegetable shortening
- ¼ cup 1% milk
- ½ cup water

Directions

- Start by preheating the oven to 350ºF.
- Take a bowl and sift dry the ingredients.
- Next step is to cut in the shortening until coarse crumbs form. Once done, make a well in the mixture.
- Now, pour the milk and water into the well.
- Stir quickly with a fork until dough follows fork around the bowl. The dough should be soft.
- Turn the dough onto lightly floured surface and knead gently for about 10 to 12 times. Roll or pat the dough until it is ½" thick.
- Now, take a 2 ½" biscuit cutter and dip it into the flour; to cut out approx. 10 biscuits.
- Finally, bake the biscuits on ungreased baking sheet for about 12 to 15 minutes.

Nutritional content per serving

Nutrition	Amount per serving
Calories	162
Trans Fat	1 gram
Sodium	150 milligrams
Protein	3 grams
Cholesterol	1 milligrams
Potassium	36 milligrams
Total Fat	8 grams
Carbohydrates	21 grams
Phosphorus	63 milligrams
Saturated Fat	2 grams
Fiber	1 gram
Calcium	92 milligrams

SIMPLY OLD STYLE PANCAKES

Yield: 4 small pancakes

Serving size: 1 pancake

Ingredients

- ½ cup all-purpose flour
- 1 egg, beaten
- ¼ cup granulated sugar
- ¼ teaspoon baking powder
- ¼ cup 2% milk plus ¼ cup water
- 1 tablespoon vegetable oil

Directions

- Take a bowl and combine the first four ingredients. Mix them well.
- Now, add water and milk. For thinner pancakes, add more water or for thicker pancakes, less water.
- Now, take a griddle or skillet and heat oil.
- Pour ¼ cup of batter on the griddle and cook until the pan cake is brown, turning on each side.

Nutritional content per serving

Nutrition	Amount per serving
Calories	165
Trans Fat	0 grams
Sodium	58 milligrams
Protein	4 grams
Cholesterol	61 milligrams
Potassium	57 milligrams
Total Fat	5 grams
Carbohydrates	26 grams
Phosphorus	64 milligrams
Saturated Fat	1 gram
Fiber	0 grams
Calcium	45 milligram

THE FRENCH TOAST

Yield: 4 servings

Serving size: 1 slice

Ingredients

- 4 large egg whites, slightly beaten
- ¼ cup 1% milk
- ½ teaspoon cinnamon
- ¼ teaspoon allspice
- 4 slices white bread (may be toasted)
- 1 tablespoon margarine

Directions

- Start by adding milk, allspice and cinnamon to the egg whites.
- Now, dip the bread into the batter, one piece at a time.
- Now, place the bread on a heated grill or in a skillet with melted margarine.
- Turn the bread once turns golden brown.
- To Serve: serve hot with sugar free syrup.

Nutritional content per serving

Nutrition	Amount per serving
Calories	125
Trans Fat	0 grams
Sodium	194 milligrams

Protein	7 grams
Cholesterol	0 milligrams
Potassium	128 milligrams
Total Fat	5 grams
Carbohydrates	14 grams
Phosphorus	61 milligrams
Saturated Fat	0 grams
Fiber	1 gram
Calcium	60 milligrams

ONIONS & CELERY BREAD DRESSING

Yield: 4 servings

Serving size: ½ cup

Ingredients

- 2 tablespoons margarine
- ¼ cup chopped onions
- 1 ½ cups plain bread crumbs or 3 slices bread, crumbled
- ¼ cup chopped celery
- 1 teaspoon poultry seasoning
- ¼ teaspoon garlic powder
- ¼ cup unsalted chicken broth

Directions

- Take a small skillet and melt margarine in it. Once the butter is melted, add the onions and sauté until the onions are tender.
- Now, add the bread crumbs, stirring constantly until crumbs get a little color.
- Now, remove the skillet from heat and add poultry seasoning, celery, garlic powder and chicken broth.
- Blend everything well and place in a small baking pan.
- Now, bake it for about 30 minutes at 375ºF.
- If the dressing appears too dry, you may add a little water as needed.

Nutritional content per serving

Nutrition	Amount per serving
Calories	107
Trans Fat	0 grams
Sodium	129 milligrams
Protein	2 grams
Cholesterol	11 milligrams
Potassium	77 milligrams
Total Fat	6 grams
Carbohydrates	11 grams
Phosphorus	30 milligrams
Saturated Fat	0 grams
Fiber	1 gram
Calcium	35 milligrams

THE DINNER ROLLS

Yield: 20 servings

Serving size: 1 roll

Ingredients

- 1 cup hot water
- 6 tablespoons vegetable shortening
- ½ cup sugar
- 1 package yeast
- 2 tablespoons of warm water
- 1 egg
- 3 ¾-4 cups all-purpose flour

Directions

- Start by preheating the oven to 400ºF.
- Take a large bowl and combine hot water, sugar and shortening. Now keep aside to cool to the room temperature.
- Now, dissolve the yeast in warm water.
- Next step is to take a large bowl and add the egg, half the flour and yeast. Beat the mixture well.
- Now, stir in remaining flour with a spoon, until it's easy to handle.
- Now, place the dough in a greased bowl; grease top and cover top with plastic wrap.
- Allow to rest for about 1 to 1 ½ hours or until the dough has doubled in size.
- Cut the amount of dough needed to shape the rolls.

• Finally, bake the rolls for about 12 minutes or until done.

Nutritional content per serving

Nutrition	Amount per serving
Calories	148
Trans Fat	0 grams
Sodium	5 milligrams
Protein	3 grams
Cholesterol	12 milligrams
Potassium	31 milligrams
Total Fat	4 grams
Carbohydrates	24 grams
Phosphorus	32 milligrams
Saturated Fat	1 grams
Fiber	1 gram
Calcium	5 milligrams

HERBS & VEGGIES RICE CASSEROLE

Yield: 8 servings

Serving size: ½ cup

Ingredients

- 1 cup white rice, uncooked
- 2 cups chicken stock, unsalted (homemade)
- ¼ cup green bell pepper, chopped
- ½ teaspoon parsley flakes
- 1 tablespoon vegetable oil
- 3 Fresh green onions, chopped
- 1 tablespoon chives

Directions

- Start by preheating the oven to 350ºF.
- Next step is to combine all the ingredients and place in casserole dish.
- Finally, bake in a covered casserole for about 45 to 50 minutes or until the liquid is absorbed.

Nutritional content per serving

Nutrition	Amount per serving
Calories	53
Trans Fat	0 grams
Sodium	19 milligrams

Protein	2 grams
Cholesterol	0 milligrams
Potassium	74 milligrams
Total Fat	2 grams
Carbohydrates	7 grams
Phosphorus	29 milligrams
Saturated Fat	0 grams
Fiber	0 grams
Calcium	7 milligrams

SIMPLE CORN PUDDING

Yield: 6 servings

Serving size: ½ cup

Ingredients

- 2 cups kernel corn, canned or fresh cut
- 3 slightly beaten eggs or ¾ cup egg substitute
- ½ cup 1% milk
- ½ cup water
- ⅓ cup onions, finely chopped
- 1 tablespoon butter, melted
- 1 teaspoon granulated sugar
- 1 teaspoon white or black pepper

Directions

- Start by preheating the oven to 350ºF.
- Take a bowl and combine all the ingredients.
- Pour the combined ingredients into a 1 ½-quart greased casserole dish.
- Place the dish in a shallow pan filled with about 1 inch of hot water.
- Bake for about 40 to 45 minutes, or until the knife inserted in center of pudding comes out clean.
- Let the pudding stand for about 10 minutes at room temperature before serving.

Nutritional content per serving

Nutrition	Amount per serving
Calories	120
Trans Fat	0 grams
Sodium	61 milligrams
Protein	6 grams
Cholesterol	121 milligrams
Potassium	234 milligrams
Total Fat	5 grams
Carbohydrates	17 grams
Phosphorus	122 milligrams
Saturated Fat	2 grams
Fiber	2 grams
Calcium	49 milligrams

Vegetables Recipes

MUSHROOMS & FRESH GREEN BEANS

Yield: 6 servings

Serving size: ½ cup

Ingredients

- 2 cans whole green beans, drained and rinsed
- 1 small onion, chopped
- ½ cup fresh mushrooms, sliced
- 1 teaspoon paprika
- ¼ teaspoon coarse black pepper
- 1 ½ cups unsalted top cracker crumbs
- 4 tablespoons margarine, unsalted

Directions

- Start by preheating the oven to 350°F.
- Take a bowl and mix together onions, green beans, mushrooms, black pepper and paprika.
- Place the mixed ingredients in a greased baking dish.
- Now, top the green beans mixture with margarine and cracker crumbs.
- Bake for about 30 to 35 minutes.

Nutritional content per serving

Nutrition	Amount per serving
Calories	137
Trans Fat	0 grams
Sodium	77 milligrams
Protein	2 grams
Cholesterol	0 milligrams
Potassium	214 milligrams
Total Fat	9 grams
Carbohydrates	14 grams
Phosphorus	38 milligrams
Saturated Fat	2 grams
Fiber	2 grams
Calcium	38 milligrams

THE MACARONI SALAD

Yield: 8 servings

Serving size: ½ cup

Ingredients

- 3 cups macaroni, cooked
- ¼ cup pimentos
- ½ cup onion, chopped
- ½ cup green pepper, chopped
- 3 hard boiled, shelled eggs, chopped
- ½ cup mayonnaise
- ½ cup celery, chopped
- 1 teaspoon dry mustard
- Paprika
- Black pepper

Directions

- Cook the macaroni as per the package directions. Once cooked, rinse the cooked macaroni under cold water and drain well.
- Now, combine the macaroni with all remaining ingredients except the black pepper and paprika. Mix everything well.
- Now, sprinkle with black pepper and paprika.
- Chill and serve.

Nutritional content per serving

Nutrition	Amount per serving
Calories	223
Trans Fat	0 grams
Sodium	103 milligrams
Protein	6 grams
Cholesterol	80 milligrams
Potassium	106 milligrams
Total Fat	14 grams
Carbohydrates	18 grams
Phosphorus	74 milligrams
Saturated Fat	2 grams
Fiber	2 grams
Calcium	20 milligrams

VEGETABLES & RICE

Yield: 6 servings

Serving size: ½ cup

Ingredients

- 2 ½ cups rice, cooked, salt-free
- 1 10-ounce package frozen green peas, cooked and drained
- 1 medium onion, chopped
- ¼ cup margarine, unsalted
- 1 tablespoon lemon juice
- ½ teaspoon thyme
- 2 tablespoons liquid smoke (optional)

Directions

- Take a pan and sauté the chopped onions in the margarine until onions are tender.
- Now, add rice, lemon juice, green peas, liquid smoke and thyme.
- Cook for about 5 minutes.

Nutritional content per serving

Nutrition	Amount per serving
Calories	194
Trans Fat	0 grams
Sodium	32 milligrams

Protein	4 grams
Cholesterol	0 milligrams
Potassium	99 milligrams
Total Fat	8 grams
Carbohydrates	26 grams
Phosphorus	67 milligrams
Saturated Fat	2 grams
Fiber	3 grams
Calcium	23 milligrams

THE COLESLAW

Yield: 4 servings

Serving size: ½ cup

Ingredients

- 1 cup cabbage, shredded
- 2 tablespoons green pepper, chopped
- ¼ cup onion, chopped
- ¼ cup carrots, shredded
- ¼ cup mayonnaise
- 2 tablespoons vinegar
- 1 tablespoon sugar
- ½ teaspoon black pepper
- ½ teaspoon celery seed (optional)
- ⅛ teaspoon dill weeds (optional)

Directions

- Start by taking a mixing bowl and combining all the vegetables.
- Take another small bowl and blend mayonnaise, seasonings and vinegar well.
- Now, pour the mayonnaise mix over the vegetables and toss.

Nutritional content per serving

Nutrition	Amount per serving
Calories	127
Trans Fat	0 grams
Sodium	81 milligrams
Protein	0 gram
Cholesterol	0 milligrams
Potassium	76 milligrams
Total Fat	11 grams
Carbohydrates	6 grams
Phosphorus	14 milligrams
Saturated Fat	2 grams
Fiber	1 gram
Calcium	13 milligrams

STEAMED FRESH ASPARAGUS

Yield: 4 servings

Serving size: 3 spears

Ingredients

- 1 tablespoon lemon juice
- 2 tablespoons margarine, melted (unsalted)
- 2 cups water
- 12 fresh asparagus spears

Directions

- Start by adding the lemon juice to the margarine and set aside.
- Now, bring the water to a boil in bottom of steamer.
- Place the asparagus in the steamer over boiling water.
- Now, steam for about 2 to 4 minutes after the asparagus turns bright green. Please make sure that the asparagus is either well or soft cooked.
- Now, remove and pour the margarine with lemon juice over asparagus and serve.

Nutritional content per serving

Nutrition	Amount per serving
Calories	62
Trans Fat	0 grams
Sodium	1 milligram
Protein	1 gram

Cholesterol	0 milligrams
Potassium	123 milligrams
Total Fat	6 grams
Carbohydrates	3 grams
Phosphorus	32 milligrams
Saturated Fat	1 gram
Fiber	1 gram
Calcium	16 milligrams

SIMPLY MARINATED VEGGIES

Yield: 15 servings

Serving size: ½ cup

Ingredients for marinade

- ¾ cup vinegar
- ¾ cup sugar
- 1 tablespoon water
- Black pepper, to taste

Ingredient for salad

- 1 12-ounce can small English peas, drained
- 1 12-ounce can shoe peg corn, drained (or normal white or yellow corn)
- 1 12-ounce jar pimento, drained
- ¾ cup onion, finely chopped
- 1 cup celery, finely chopped

Directions

- Take a small saucepan and combine the marinade ingredients and bring them to a boil. Once boiled, cool completely.
- Take another bowl and mix the salad ingredients together.
- Now, pour cooled marinade over the vegetables and stir well.
- Finally, place it in a covered container and then refrigerate overnight before serving.

Nutritional content per serving

Nutrition	Amount per serving
Calories	85
Trans Fat	0 grams
Sodium	13 milligrams
Protein	1 gram
Cholesterol	0 milligrams
Potassium	154 milligrams
Total Fat	0 grams
Carbohydrates	20 grams
Phosphorus	39 milligrams
Saturated Fat	0 grams
Fiber	2 grams
Calcium	12 milligrams

THE GREEN SALAD

Yield: 6 cups

Serving size: 1 cup

Ingredients

- 4 cups red leaf or other lettuce, shredded
- 1 carrot, sliced
- 2 celery stalks, sliced
- 2 cucumbers, sliced
- 2 radishes, sliced
- 1 large bell pepper, diced or sliced into rings

Directions

- Take a large bowl and combine the vegetables and toss well.
- You may serve this salad with your favorite salad dressings.

Nutritional content per serving

Nutrition	Amount per serving
Calories	30
Trans Fat	0 grams
Sodium	20 milligrams
Protein	1 gram
Cholesterol	0 milligrams
Potassium	215 milligrams
Total Fat	0 grams
Carbohydrates	4 grams

Phosphorus	29 milligrams
Saturated Fat	0 grams
Fiber	1 gram
Calcium	25 milligrams

SPRING ONIONS & SQUASH

Yield: 3 servings

Serving size: ½ cup

Ingredients

- 2 cups yellow straight neck or crook neck squash, washed and sliced
- 2 tablespoons butter or margarine
- 1 cup green onion, chopped
- 1 teaspoon black pepper

Directions

- Start by boiling the squash slices for about 15 minutes or until tender. Drain.
- Take a frying pan and melt the butter. Sauté the spring onions for about one minute.
- Now, stir in the squash and black pepper.
- Cover the pan and allow it to simmer on low heat for about 5 minutes.
- Serve hot.

Nutritional content per serving

Nutrition	Amount per serving
Calories	87
Trans Fat	1 gram
Sodium	347 milligrams
Protein	1.5 gram
Cholesterol	0 milligrams
Potassium	204 milligrams
Total Fat	8 grams
Carbohydrates	4 grams
Phosphorus	40 milligrams
Saturated Fat	2 grams
Fiber	2 grams
Calcium	31 milligrams

OVEN BAKED YELLOW SQUASH

Yield: 6 servings

Serving size: ½ cup

Ingredients

- 2 tablespoons margarine or butter, melted
- ¾ teaspoon thyme
- ⅛ teaspoon black pepper
- 2 cans yellow squash, sliced
- 1 medium onion, chopped
- 1 small stalk celery, chopped
- 1 large bell pepper, chopped
- 1 tablespoon lemon juice

Directions

- Start by preheating the oven to 350°F.
- Next step is to sauté all the ingredients except the lemon juice in margarine. Cook until the onions become translucent.
- Now, add the lemon juice.
- Now, place the sautéed mixture in a casserole dish.
- Finally, bake it for about 30 minutes.
- Serve hot.

Nutritional content per serving

Nutrition	Amount per serving
Calories	49
Trans Fat	1 gram
Sodium	34 milligrams
Protein	1 grams
Cholesterol	0 milligrams
Potassium	139 milligrams
Total Fat	3 grams
Carbohydrates	5 grams
Phosphorus	25 milligrams
Saturated Fat	1 gram
Fiber	2 grams
Calcium	31 milligrams

FRIED ONION RINGS

Yield: 10 servings

Serving size: 7 rings

Ingredients

- ¾ cup plain cornmeal
- ¼ cup all-purpose flour
- 1 teaspoon sugar
- 4 medium onions
- 1 egg, beaten
- ¼ cup water
- ½ cup vegetable oil for frying

Directions

- Start by mixing the flour, cornmeal and sugar together. Once done, keep aside.
- Now, peel the onions and cut them crosswise for about ¼" thick. Once cut, separate the onion into rings.
- Now, mix the water and beaten egg.
- Dip the onion rings in the egg wash, then into the cornmeal mixture.
- Now, fry the onion rings for about 3 to 5 minutes in hot vegetable oil, turning until brown.
- Once fried, drain the onion rings on paper towels and serve hot.

Nutritional content per serving

Nutrition	Amount per serving
Calories	162
Trans Fat	0 grams
Sodium	11 milligrams
Protein	2 grams
Cholesterol	27 milligrams
Potassium	99 milligrams
Total Fat	11 grams
Carbohydrates	14 grams
Phosphorus	39 milligrams
Saturated Fat	1 gram
Fiber	2 grams
Calcium	11 milligrams

Sauces Recipes

SWEET & NO SALT BROWN MUSTARD

Yield: 1 ½ cups

Serving size: 1 tablespoon

Ingredients

- 2 teaspoons cornstarch
- 1 cup cider vinegar
- ½ cup dry mustard
- ½ cup light brown sugar
- ½ teaspoon white pepper (or black pepper)

Directions

- Start by dissolving the corn starch in small amount of vinegar.
- Take a pan and heat the remaining vinegar. Once heated, add mustard, pepper and sugar. Stir well until sugar is dissolved.
- Once the sugar is dissolved, add the corn starch and cook until the mix becomes thick. Once the mix is thick, remove from the heat.
- Now, cover the mixture and let it stand at room temperature for about 24 hours in order to develop the flavour.

Nutritional content per serving

Nutrition	Amount per serving
Calories	27
Trans Fat	0 grams
Sodium	2 milligrams
Protein	0 grams
Cholesterol	0 milligrams
Potassium	27 milligrams
Total Fat	1 grams
Carbohydrates	4 grams
Phosphorus	18 milligrams
Saturated Fat	0 grams
Fiber	0 grams
Calcium	9 milligrams

SIMPLE HOMEMADE RELISH

Yield: 2 ¼ cups

Serving size: 1 tablespoon

Ingredients

- 2 lemons, peeled and quartered
- 1 large onion
- ½ medium green pepper
- 2 cups sliced celery
- ¼ cup parsley (optional)
- ½ cup sugar
- ¼ teaspoon ground mustard
- ⅛ teaspoon allspice
- 1 teaspoon celery seed

Directions

- Start by chopping the first five ingredients. Once chopped, stir in the spices and sugar.
- Now, cover and place in the refrigerator for overnight or several hours so that the flavors can blend.

Nutritional content per serving

Nutrition	Amount per serving
Calories	8
Trans Fat	0 grams
Sodium	8 milligrams
Protein	0 grams
Cholesterol	0 milligrams
Potassium	31 milligrams
Total Fat	0 grams
Carbohydrates	2 grams
Phosphorus	9 milligrams
Saturated Fat	0 grams
Fiber	0 grams
Calcium	10 milligrams

Chapter 9

Recipes: Beverages

A MESSAGE FOR READERS

This is important to understand that controlling your potassium intake is completely in your hands. In this chapter, you may see some recipes with more than 121-250 mg potassium per serving which is fine as you should only eat one portion of the recipe and a maximum of 2000 to 2500 milligrams of potassium per day. As long as your potassium intake is under the above mentioned limits, you will be fine.

STRAWBERRY & LEMON SORBET

Yield: 2 ½ cups

Serving size: 6-ounces or ¾ cups

Ingredients

- ¼ cup sugar
- 1 cup frozen or fresh strawberries, cleaned,
- 1 tablespoon lemon juice
- ¼ cup water
- 1 ¼ cups crushed or cubed ice

Directions

- Start by taking a blender and placing ice in it.
- Now, add all the other ingredients.
- Now, blend, liquefy or crush as per your taste and requirements.

Nutritional content per serving

Nutrition	Amount per serving
Calories	67
Trans Fat	0 grams
Sodium	1 milligrams
Protein	0 grams
Cholesterol	0 milligrams
Potassium	79 milligrams
Total Fat	16 grams

Carbohydrates	21 grams
Phosphorus	12 milligrams
Saturated Fat	0 grams
Fiber	1 gram
Calcium	9 milligrams

INSTANT RUSSIAN TEA

Yield: 5 ½ cups dry powder/88 servings

Serving size: 1 tablespoon

Ingredients

- 2 cups Tang®
- ½ cup sugar
- 1 dry lemonade mix (2 quart size)
- 1 cup instant tea
- 1 teaspoon cloves
- 1 teaspoon cinnamon

Directions

- Start by combining all the ingredients.
- Store the combined ingredients in a covered container.
- To prepare: add one tablespoon of the mix to about 8-ounces of hot water.
- Serve hot.

Nutritional content per serving

Nutrition	Amount per serving
Calories	54
Trans Fat	0 grams
Sodium	0 milligrams
Protein	0 grams
Cholesterol	0 milligrams

Potassium	25 milligrams
Total Fat	0 grams
Carbohydrates	13 grams
Phosphorus	17 milligrams
Saturated Fat	0 grams
Fiber	0 grams
Calcium	35 milligrams

HAWAIIAN PUNCH

Yield: ½ gallon or 8 servings

Serving size: 8-ounces or 1 cup

Ingredients

- 1 48-ounce can Hawaiian Punch®
- 1 32-ounce bottle ginger ale

Directions

- Combine all the ingredients and pour over the ice.
- Garnish with lime slices or lemon.

Nutritional content per serving

Nutrition	Amount per serving
Calories	103
Trans Fat	0 grams
Sodium	63 milligrams
Protein	1 gram
Cholesterol	0 milligrams
Potassium	47 milligrams
Total Fat	0 grams
Carbohydrates	26 grams
Phosphorus	5 milligrams
Saturated Fat	0 grams
Fiber	0 grams
Calcium	15 milligrams

THE JUICY PUNCH

Yield: 46 servings

Serving size: 6-ounces or ¾ cups

Ingredients

- 3 quarts cranberry juice
- 3 quarts pineapple juice
- 1 quart lemonade, frozen, undiluted
- 1 quart water
- 3 28-ounce bottles ginger ale

Directions

- Start by mixing all the ingredients together.
- Once mixed, chill in the refrigerator.
- Serve.

Nutritional content per serving

Nutrition	Amount per serving
Calories	130
Trans Fat	0 grams
Sodium	8 milligrams
Protein	1 grams
Cholesterol	0 milligrams
Potassium	153 milligrams
Total Fat	0 grams
Carbohydrates	34 grams

Phosphorus	16 milligrams
Saturated Fat	0 grams
Fiber	0 grams
Calcium	17 milligrams

SPICED UP APPLE JUICE

Yield: 8 servings

Serving size: ½ cup

Ingredients

- ½ teaspoon nutmeg
- 12 whole cloves
- 4 cinnamon sticks, broken
- ¼ teaspoon allspice
- 1 quart unsweetened apple

Directions

- Take a saucepan and place all the ingredients in it.
- Now, slowly bring it to a boil and let it simmer for about 20 minutes.
- To serve: strain the mix and serve in cups.

Nutritional content per serving

Nutrition	Amount per serving
Calories	63
Trans Fat	0 grams
Sodium	6 milligrams
Protein	1 grams
Cholesterol	0 milligrams
Potassium	132 milligrams
Total Fat	1 grams

Carbohydrates	15 grams
Phosphorus	10 milligrams
Saturated Fat	0 grams
Fiber	1 gram
Calcium	18 milligrams

Chapter 10

Recipes: Desserts

A MESSAGE FOR READERS

This is important to understand that controlling your potassium intake is completely in your hands. In this chapter, you will find deserts under 150 mg per serving. You may eat either one or two portions of such recipes but in moderation. You must not exceed the intake of potassium more than 2000 to 2500 milligrams per day. As long as your potassium intake is under the above mentioned limits, you will be fine.

FROZEN BERRY FANTASY

Yield: 4 servings

Serving size: 4-ounces

Ingredients

- 1 cup cranberry juice cocktail
- 1 cup fresh whole strawberries, washed and hulled
- 2 tablespoons fresh lime juice
- ¼ cup sugar
- 8-9 ice cubes
- Strawberries for garnishing

Directions

- Take a blender and combine strawberries, cranberry juice, sugar and lime juice.
- Now, add the ice cubes and blend until smooth.
- To serve: pour it into the chilled glasses and garnish with fresh strawberry.

Nutritional content per serving

Nutrition	Amount per serving
Calories	100
Trans Fat	0 grams
Sodium	3 milligrams
Protein	0 gram
Cholesterol	0 milligrams

Potassium	109 milligrams
Total Fat	0 gram
Carbohydrates	24 grams
Phosphorus	129 milligrams
Saturated Fat	0 gram
Fiber	1 gram
Calcium	9 milligrams

HOMEMADE RIBBON CAKES/COOKIES

Yield: 84 cookies

Serving size: 2 cookies

Ingredients

- 3 cups unsifted all-purpose flour
- 1 cup sugar
- 1 teaspoon baking powder
- 1 cup (½ pound) butter or margarine, softened
- 2 whole eggs plus 1 egg white
- ½ teaspoon vanilla
- 1 cup jelly or jam (plum, blackberry, or raspberry jelly)
- 2 tablespoons sugar

Directions

- Start by preheating the oven to 375°F.
- Take a large bowl and combine the flour, sugar, and baking powder.
- Now, blend in the butter with finger tips until mixture resembles the cornmeal.
- Now, add the egg whites, eggs and vanilla. Let's now work it into stiff dough.
- Next step is to divide the dough into two balls, one ball twice the size of the other ball. Take a heavily floured board (about

¼ to ½ cup flour) and roll out the larger ball to 1/8 inches thickness.

- Now, place the rolled dough in a cookie pan (11" x 15 ½"), smoothing out to edges and patching corners. Now, spread the jelly over the top.

- Roll out the remaining dough to 1/8 inches thickness and cut into ½ inches wide strips; place the strips diagonally across the jelly, ½ inches apart. Sprinkle sugar over the top and Place in the oven.

- When the edges start to brown (this will take about 20 minutes), take the pan from the oven, cut of and remove about a 3 inches strip all around the edges. Return the pan to the oven, remove after 10 minutes.

- Cut into 1" x 2" rectangles. Makes 7 dozen cookies.

Nutritional content per serving

Nutrition	Amount per serving
Calories	106
Trans Fat	1 gram
Sodium	65 milligrams
Protein	1 gram
Cholesterol	14 milligrams
Potassium	17 milligrams
Total Fat	5 gram
Carbohydrates	15 grams
Phosphorus	27 milligrams
Saturated Fat	1 gram
Fiber	0 grams
Calcium	11 milligrams

EGGS CUSTARD

Yield: 4 servings

Serving size: ½ cup

Ingredients

- 2 medium eggs
- ¼ cup 2% milk
- 3 tablespoons sugar
- 1 teaspoon vanilla or lemon extract
- 1 teaspoon nutmeg

Directions

- Start by preheating the oven to 325°F.
- In an electric mixer, combine all the ingredients, and beat for about one minute until the mixture is thoroughly mixed.
- Now, pour the mixture into the muffin pans or custard cups.
- Sprinkle the nutmeg on top.
- Finally, bake for about 20 to 30 minutes or until a knife inserted into the center of the custard comes out absolutely clean.

Nutritional content per serving

Nutrition	Amount per serving
Calories	70
Trans Fat	0 grams
Sodium	34 milligrams
Protein	3 grams
Cholesterol	91 milligrams
Potassium	30 milligrams
Total Fat	3 grams
Carbohydrates	9 grams
Phosphorus	42 milligrams
Saturated Fat	1 gram
Fiber	0 gram
Calcium	12 milligrams

HOMEMADE PINEAPPLE PUDDING

Yield: 12 servings

Serving size: ½ cup

Ingredients

- 3 tablespoons all-purpose flour
- ½ cup sugar
- 1 large egg, whole
- 3 large eggs, divided
- 1 cup 2% milk
- 1 cup water
- 1 teaspoon vanilla extract
- 2 cups pineapple chunks, drained
- ¼ cup sugar
- 25-30 vanilla wafers

Directions

- Start by preheating the oven to 425°F.
- Combine flour, 1 whole egg, sugar and 3 egg yolks in top of a double boiler.
- Now, stir in water and milk. Cook it uncovered over the boiling water, stirring constantly, until it thickens.
- Once thickens, remove from the heat and add vanilla extract.
- Take a 1 ½ quart casserole dish and spread a small amount of custard on the bottom. Now, top with half of the vanilla wafers, then half of the pineapple.

- Continue with the layers of custard, vanilla wafers, and pineapple, beginning and ending with the custard.
- Now, beat the remaining egg whites with a fork, hand mixer or egg beater and add sugar. Beat the egg whites until stiff peaks form.
- Now, pile the beaten egg whites on top of layered pudding.
- Finally, bake for about 5 minutes or until lightly browned.

Nutritional content per serving

Nutrition	Amount per serving
Calories	209
Trans Fat	0 grams
Sodium	80 milligrams
Protein	4 grams
Cholesterol	81 milligrams
Potassium	120 milligrams
Total Fat	5 grams
Carbohydrates	38 grams
Phosphorus	71 milligrams
Saturated Fat	2 grams
Fiber	1 gram
Calcium	47 milligrams

LEMONY COOKIES

Yield: 5 dozen

Serving size: 2 cookies

Ingredients

- 1 cup unsalted butter or margarine
- 1 cup granulated sugar
- 1 egg
- 1 ½ teaspoons lemon extract
- 1 ½ cup all-purpose flour, sifted

Directions

- Start by preheating the oven to 375°F.
- Next step is to cream the butter with sugar.
- Now, add the egg, lemon extract and beat until it is light and fluffy.
- Now, add the flour and mix until it is smooth.
- It's now time to drop the batter by level tablespoon onto the ungreased cookie sheet. Maintain a distance between the cookies of at least 2".
- Finally, bake the cookies for about 10 minutes or until the cookies brown around the edges.
- Once done, cool for a minute and remove the cookies from the cookie sheet.

Nutritional content per serving

Nutrition	Amount per serving
Calories	115
Trans Fat	0 grams
Sodium	12 milligrams
Protein	2 gram
Cholesterol	76 milligrams
Potassium	20 milligrams
Total Fat	6 grams
Carbohydrates	12 grams
Phosphorus	23 milligrams
Saturated Fat	1 gram
Fiber	0 grams
Calcium	7 milligrams

GUMDROPS COOKIES

Yield: 50 cookies

Serving size: 2 cookies

Ingredients

- ½ cup softened unsalted butter or margarine
- 1 cup brown sugar, packed
- 1 medium egg
- ¼ cup milk
- 1 teaspoon vanilla
- 1 ¾ cups all-purpose flour, sifted
- 1 teaspoon baking powder
- 15 large gumdrops, chopped

Directions

- Start by preheating the oven to 400°F.
- Next step is to cream the butter, egg and sugar thoroughly.
- Now, stir in the vanilla and milk.
- Take another bowl and mix the flour with baking powder. Once mixed, add flour and baking powder mix to the above ingredients.
- Now, add and mix in the gumdrops and chill the dough for at least 1 hour.
- Now, drop the dough by tablespoonful onto the greased cookie sheet.
- Finally, bake for about 8 to 10 minutes or until the cookies are golden brown.

Nutritional content per serving

Nutrition	Amount per serving
Calories	104
Trans Fat	0 grams
Sodium	9 milligrams
Protein	1 gram
Cholesterol	7 milligrams
Potassium	29 milligrams
Total Fat	1 gram
Carbohydrates	22 grams
Phosphorus	16 milligrams
Saturated Fat	0 grams
Fiber	0 grams
Calcium	13 milligrams

VANILLA ALMOND FLAVORED COOKIES

Yield: 75 cookies

Serving size: 2 cookies

Ingredients

- 5 cups all-purpose flour
- 2 cups butter
- 1 cup plus 2 tablespoons sugar
- 2 eggs
- 1 teaspoon almond extract
- 2 teaspoons vanilla extract

Directions

- Start by preheating the oven to 400°F.
- Next step is to combine the flour, sugar and butter.
- Now, add eggs, vanilla extract, almond extract and mix with a hand mixer on low speed or spoon.
- Now, drop the cookies onto the ungreased baking sheet. You can also use a cookie gun to drop the batter.
- Finally, bake for about 5 to 8 minutes.
- Cool before serve.

Nutritional content per serving

Nutrition	Amount per serving
Calories	172
Trans Fat	0 grams
Sodium	56 milligrams
Protein	2 grams
Cholesterol	13 milligrams
Potassium	29 milligrams
Total Fat	7 grams
Carbohydrates	26 grams
Phosphorus	22 milligrams
Saturated Fat	4 grams
Fiber	0 grams
Calcium	8 milligrams

THE POUND CAKE

Yield: 24 servings

Serving size: 1 slice (3 ½" x 4" x ¾")

Ingredients

- 2 cups butter or margarine
- 4 cups powdered sugar
- 2 tablespoons grated lemon rind
- 1 teaspoon lemon extract
- 6 eggs
- 3 ½ cups all-purpose flour, sifted

Directions

- Start by preheating the oven to 350°F.
- In an electric mixer, cream the butter for about 3 minutes on medium speed, or until it is light and fluffy.
- Then gradually add the sugar, lemon rind and cream the mixture thoroughly.
- Now, add the eggs and lemon extract, one at a time. Mix well after each addition.
- Gradually add the flour and mix well.
- Now, pour the mix into the greased and floured 10 inches Bundt pan or tube pan.
- Now, bake for about 1 hour and 20 minutes or until a wooden pick inserted in center of pound cake comes out absolutely clean.
- Remove the cake from the pan.

- Cool and serve.

Nutritional content per serving

Nutrition	Amount per serving
Calories	279
Trans Fat	0 grams
Sodium	127 milligrams
Protein	10 grams
Cholesterol	267 milligrams
Potassium	108 milligrams
Total Fat	11 grams
Carbohydrates	34 grams
Phosphorus	139 milligrams
Saturated Fat	5 grams
Fiber	0 grams
Calcium	40 milligram

HOMEMADE PINEAPPLE POUND CAKE

Yield: 24 servings

Serving size: 1 slice (3 ½" x 4" x ¾")

Ingredients for cake

- 3 cups sugar
- 1 ½ cups butter
- 6 whole eggs and 4 egg whites
- 1 teaspoon vanilla extract
- 3 cups all-purpose flour, sifted
- 1 10-ounce can crushed pineapple (drain and reserve juice)

Ingredients for glaze

- 1 cup sugar
- 1 stick margarine (½ cup)
- Juice from pineapple

Directions

- Start by preheating the oven to 350°F.
- Next step is to beat together the butter and sugar until the mixture becomes smooth and creamy.
- Then add the eggs whites and eggs, two at a time, mixing after each addition.

- Then add the vanilla extract.
- Then add the sifted flour and mix well.
- Then add the drained and crushed pineapple.
- Now, bake for about 45 minutes to 1 hour.
- While it bakes, take a medium saucepan and mix together the ingredients for glaze.
- Bring to a boil, stirring frequently, until the desired thickness is reached.
- Finally, pour it over the top of the cake while it's still hot.

Nutritional content per serving

Nutrition	Amount per serving
Calories	288
Trans Fat	0 grams
Sodium	93 milligrams
Protein	2. 5 grams
Cholesterol	68 milligrams
Potassium	67 milligrams
Total Fat	9 grams
Carbohydrates	47 grams
Phosphorus	47 milligrams
Saturated Fat	6 grams
Fiber	19 grams
Calcium	19 milligrams

HOMEMADE WHIPPED CREAM POUND CAKE

Yield: 30 slices

Serving size: 1 slice

Ingredients

- 2 sticks margarine or butter, softened
- 3 cups sugar
- 6 eggs
- 3 cups cake flour (sift once before measuring)
- ½ pint whipping cream
- 1 teaspoon vanilla flavoring

Directions

- Start by preheating the oven to 350°F.
- Take a tube pan, grease and flour it.
- Please make sure that all the ingredients of this recipe should be at room temperature.
- Next step is to cream the margarine and sugar until fluffy.
- Now, add the eggs, one at a time, beating after each addition.
- Then, gradually add the flour and whipping cream, blending between each addition.
- Beat the mixture well for about 30 seconds and then stir in the vanilla flavoring.
- Finally, pour the batter into the tube pan and bake for about 50 to 60 minutes.

Nutritional content per serving

Nutrition	Amount per serving
Calories	249
Trans Fat	0 grams
Sodium	192 milligrams
Protein	8 grams
Cholesterol	6 milligrams
Potassium	120 milligrams
Total Fat	9 grams
Carbohydrates	35 grams
Phosphorus	24 milligrams
Saturated Fat	2.5 grams
Fiber	0 grams
Calcium	12 milligrams

THE SPICED UP POUND CAKE

Yield: 16 slices

Serving size: 1 slice

Ingredients

- 3 sticks butter or margarine
- 1 ¼teaspoons ground nutmeg or mace
- 1 teaspoon vanilla extract
- 1 pound sifted powdered sugar
- 6 eggs
- 3 cups cake flour
- Powdered sugar

Directions

- Start by preheating the oven to 325°F.
- Next step is to take a large bowl and cream the butter until softened.
- Now, blend in the vanilla extract and nutmeg.
- Then gradually stir in the powdered sugar.
- Add the eggs, one at a time, beating well after each addition.
- Then gradually stir in the flour.
- Take a 10" x 4" round tube pan, grease only the bottom and flour it lightly. Note: please do not grease the sides of the tube pan.
- Now, bake for about 1 hour and 20 minutes or until a cake tester inserted in the center comes out absolutely clean.
- Once done, allow the cake to cool.

- Once cool, sprinkle with the powdered sugar, cut and serve.

Nutritional content per serving

Nutrition	Amount per serving
Calories	174
Trans Fat	0 grams
Sodium	45 milligrams
Protein	3 grams
Cholesterol	82 milligrams
Potassium	51 milligrams
Total Fat	5 grams
Carbohydrates	33 grams
Phosphorus	25 milligrams
Saturated Fat	2 grams
Fiber	0 grams
Calcium	7 milligrams

CHUNKY PINEAPPLE CAKE

Yield: 20 Squares

Serving size: 1 square

Ingredients

- 2 sticks margarine
- 2 ½ cups sugar
- 1 teaspoons vanilla extract
- 4 eggs
- 4 egg whites
- 3 cups all-purpose flour, sifted
- ½ cup butter or margarine
- 1 16-ounce can crushed pineapple, drained
- ¾ cup brown sugar

Directions

- Start by preheating the oven to 375°F.
- In an electric mixer, cream the margarine until it is light and fluffy. Gradually add the sugar and cream the mix thoroughly.
- Now, add the vanilla extract, eggs whites and eggs, two at a time.
- Then gradually add the flour and mix well.
- Take a cake pan and melt ½ cup of butter.
- Once melted, spread the pineapple evenly in the pan and sprinkle the brown sugar over pineapple.
- Now, pour the batter over pineapple and bake for about 45 minutes.

- When done, turn the cake over onto a cake plate.
- Slice and serve.

Nutritional content per serving

Nutrition	Amount per serving
Calories	301
Trans Fat	0 grams
Sodium	123 milligrams
Protein	4 grams
Cholesterol	206 milligrams
Potassium	76 milligrams
Total Fat	9 grams
Carbohydrates	53 grams
Phosphorus	26 milligrams
Saturated Fat	3 grams
Fiber	1 gram
Calcium	43 milligrams

APPLES CRUNCH

Yield: 8 servings

Serving size: ½ cup

Ingredients

- 4 large tart apples, pared, cored and sliced
- ¾ cup sugar
- ½ cups all-purpose flour, sifted
- ⅓ cup margarine, softened
- ¾ cup rolled oats
- ¾ teaspoon nutmeg

Directions

- Start by preheating the oven to 375°F.
- Place the apples in a greased 8 inches square pan.
- Take a medium bowl and combine the remaining ingredients and spread over apples.
- Finally, bake for about 30 to 35 minutes or until the apples are tender and lightly browned.

Nutritional content per serving

Nutrition	Amount per serving
Calories	217
Trans Fat	1.4 grams
Sodium	62 milligrams

Protein	1.4 grams
Cholesterol	0 milligrams
Potassium	68 milligrams
Total Fat	2 grams
Carbohydrates	36 grams
Phosphorus	37 milligrams
Saturated Fat	2 grams
Fiber	2 grams
Calcium	10 milligrams

FREEZE IT LEMON

Yield: 8 squares

Serving size: 1 square

Ingredients

- 4 eggs, separated
- ⅔ cup sugar
- ¼ cup lemon juice
- 1 tablespoon lemon peel, grated
- 1 cup whipping cream, whipped
- 2 cups vanilla wafers (about 40), crushed

Directions

- Start by beating the egg yolks until very thick.
- Then gradually beat in the sugar. Beat well after each addition.
- Now, add the lemon peel, lemon juice and blend well.
- It's time now to cook the mix in a double boiler over hot water stirring constantly until thick.
- Once cooked, remove it from the heat and allow cooling.
- Now, beat the egg whites until stiff peaks form.
- Now, fold in the egg whites into cooled thickened mixture.
- Now, fold in the whipped cream.
- Now, take a freezer tray or a 10" x 6" x 1 ½" baking dish and spread 1 and half cups of vanilla wafer crumbs in the bottom.
- Now, spoon the lemon mixture all over the crumbs.
- Now, top with the remaining vanilla wafer crumbs.
- Finally, freeze it for overnight or several hours or until firm.

Nutritional content per serving

Nutrition	Amount per serving
Calories	205
Trans Fat	0 grams
Sodium	97 milligrams
Protein	3 grams
Cholesterol	27 milligrams
Potassium	69 milligrams
Total Fat	7 grams
Carbohydrates	32 grams
Phosphorus	33 milligrams
Saturated Fat	4 grams
Fiber	0 grams
Calcium	22 milligrams

End of Recipes

Wrapping Up!

What you eat and drink can help slow down and cure you. Some foods are better for you than others. Cooking and preparing your food from scratch and fresh at home can help you eat healthier. Always read the specified nutritional values per servings and try to eat not more than one portion of recommended servings.

To help control your sodium level in the body, try to use alternatives to the salt as suggested in the book. Limit the intake of phosphorus and potassium to recommended amounts. Eat the right amount and right type of protein, especially from high quality sources of protein like eggs, poultry, red meat, seafood and milk (*Though milk is high in potassium but can be used in moderation*).

At last, I would like to thank you for reading this book and hope that you will create a new healthier you!

RECIPES INDEX

34574527R10112

Made in the USA
Middletown, DE
26 August 2016